PLAB 2
Made Easy

OSCEs with discussion

Elora Mukherjee MBBS MRCP
King's College Hospital, London

Edited by
Jonathan Treml MBBS BA MRCP
Consultant Geriatrician
Selly Oak Hospital, Birmingham

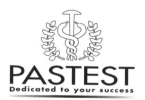

PASTEST
Dedicated to your success

© 2003 PASTEST Ltd
Egerton Court
Parkgate Estate
Knutsford
Cheshire
WA16 8DX

Telephone: 01565 752000

First published 2003
Reprinted 2006

ISBN: 1 901198 92 8

A catalogue record for this book is available from the British Library.

The information contained within this book was obtained by the authors from reliable sources. However, while every effort has been made to ensure its accuracy, no responsibility for loss, damage or injury occasioned to any person acting or refraining from action as a result of information contained herein can be accepted by the publishers or authors.

PasTest Revision Books and Intensive Courses

PasTest has been established in the field of postgraduate medical education since 1972, providing revision books and intensive study courses for doctors preparing for their professional examinations. Books and courses are available for the following specialties:

MRCGP, MRCP Part 1 and 2, MRCPCH Part 1 and 2, MRCPsych, MRCS, MRCOG, DRCOG, DCH, FRCA, PLAB.

For further details contact:

PasTest, Freepost, Knutsford, Cheshire WA16 7BR
Tel: 01565 752000 Fax: 01565 650264
www.pastest.co.uk   enquiries@pastest.co.uk

Cover design by Taylor Moore Graphics
Text prepared by Vision Typesetting, Manchester
Printed and bound in Great Britain by Page Bros (Norwich) Ltd

Contents

Foreword

Congratulations! If you are reading this then, hopefully, you have already passed Part 1 and are well on the way to completing the final hurdle before being able to work as a doctor in the UK. The good news is that PLAB Part 2 is a clinical exam. This means that it should be testing knowledge, skills and attitudes that you have already put into practice as a doctor elsewhere. This book will not teach you how to be a doctor, nor will it even teach you the basics of clinical skills as there are already many books that serve this purpose. The content is purposely designed to provide a format and structure to revise for the specific challenges of the PLAB Part 2 exam. In particular, it provides a framework for the commonest clinical procedures that are tested and a number of examples of exam stations that test communication skills.

Good communication skills are essential for passing PLAB. The reason for this is obvious – to be a good doctor, you must be a good communicator. Testing communication is not just a matter of assessing written and spoken English – you will already have demonstrated this in a previous exam. Communication is about the whole process of talking and listening, the giving and eliciting of information.

A selection of scenarios are provided where these essential skills are demonstrated with examples of good practice. However, you cannot expect to pass the exam just by reading this book. It is vital that you put these skills into practice on a regular basis. Ask family, friends and colleagues to pretend that they are patients and practise taking a history from them (remembering that the clock is always running). You will also be able to come up with additional scenarios of your own. You must also practise giving information, taking consent, counselling and breaking bad news. All of these skills should already be familiar to you but there is always room for improvement.

Enjoy working your way through the book and GOOD LUCK.

Jonathan Treml

List of contributors

Adrian Alexander Boyle BM MRCP M.Phil
Health Services Research Fellow and Honorary Specialist Registrar
in Emergency Medicine, Department of Psychiatry,
Addenbrooke's Hospital, Cambridge.

Jayanta Chatterjee MBBS, DFFP
Clinical Fellow with special interest in Infertility, Department of
Obstetrics and Gynaecology, Fertility Unit,
St Bartholomew's Hospital, London.

Anthony Gallagher MBBS
Locum Specialist Registrar, Accident and Emergency Department,
Peterborough District Hospital, Peterborough.

Soumyen Maitra MBBS, FRCS
Staff Grade, Accident & Emergency Department,
Countess of Chester Hospital, Chester.

Tapas Mukherjee
5th year Medical Student, Manchester Royal Infirmary, Manchester.

I would like to dedicate this book to Bani and Rabin Mukherjee, my mother and father.

Acknowledgement

The author and publishers would like to acknowledge Peterborough District Hospital, Clinical Skills Laboratory, Post Graduate Medical Centre who have kindly given us permission to reproduce colour images on the following pages: 197, 201, 207, 213, 214, 215, 225, 228, 229, 231, 239.

List of abbreviations

A&E	Accident and Emergency (department)
AA	Alcoholics Anonymous
ABC	airway, breathing, circulation
ABG	arterial blood gas
ACE	angiotensin-converting enzyme
AF	atrial fibrillation
ALP	alkaline phosphatase
ALT	alanine aminotransferase
AST	aspartate aminotransferase
AV	atrioventricular
AVPU	Alert, Verbal, Painful, Unresponsive (scale)
bd/bid	*bis die* (i.e. twice a day)
BLS	basic life support
BM	basal metabolism
BNF	*British National Formulary*
BP	blood pressure
BTS	British Thoracic Society
CCU	coronary/cardiac care unit
COPD	chronic obstructive pulmonary disease
CP	cerebral palsy
CPAP	continuous positive airways pressure
CPN	community psychiatric nurse
CPR	cardiopulmonary resuscitation
CRAO	central retinal artery occlusion
CRVO	central retinal vein occlusion
CT	computed tomography
CVS	chorionic villous sampling
CXR	chest X-ray

D&C	dilatation and curettage
dL	decilitre (i.e. 100 ml)
DSH	deliberate self-harm
DVLA	Driver and Vehicle Licensing Agency
DVT	deep vein thrombosis
EBV	Epstein–Barr virus
EC	emergency contraceptive
ECG	electrocardiogram/graphy
EDTA	ethylenediamine tetra-acetic acid
ELISA	enzyme-linked immunosorbent assay
F	French (catheter gauge)
FBC	full blood count
FEV_1	forced expired volume of air in 1 s
fL	femtolitre (i.e. 10^{-15} litres)
FNA	fine-needle aspiration
FSH	follicle-stimulating hormone
FVC	forced vital capacity
GCS	Glasgow Coma Scale
GI	gastrointestinal
GMC	General Medical Council
GP	general practitioner
GTN	glyceryl trinitrate
GUM	genitourinary medicine
h	hour
Hb	haemoglobin
Hb A_{1C}	haemoglobin A_{1C}
HIV	human immunodeficiency virus
HPO	hypothalamic-pituitary-ovarian (axis)
HRT	hormone-replacement therapy
HSP	Henoch–Schönlein purpura
ICE	Ideas, Concerns, Expectations
ID	identity
IDA	iron deficiency anaemia
IDDM	insulin-dependent diabetes mellitus
IHD	ischaemic heart disease
im	intramuscular

INR	international normalised ratio
ITU	intensive therapy unit
IUCD	intrauterine contraceptive device
iv	intravenous
IVDA	intravenous drug abuse
IVF	*in vitro* fertilisation
JVP	jugular venous pulse
L	litre
LDL	low-density lipoprotein
LFT	lung function test
LH	luteinising hormone
LMP	last menstrual period
LSD	lysergic acid diethylamide
LTOT	long-term oxygen therapy
LVF	left ventricular failure
MCH	mean corpuscular haemoglobin
MCHC	mean corpuscular haemoglobin concentration
MCV	mean corpuscular volume
μg	microgram (10^{-6} grams, i.e. one-millionth of a gram)
mg	milligram (10^{-3}, i.e. one-thousandth of a gram)
MHAT	mental health assessment team
MI	myocardial infarct(ion)
min	minute
ml	millilitre (i.e. 10^{-3} litres)
mmol/L	millimoles/litre (i.e. 10^{-3} moles/litre)
MTPJs	metatarsophalangeal joints
mV	millivolt
NIDDM	non-insulin-dependent diabetes mellitus
NSAID	non-steroidal anti-inflammatory drug
od	once a day
OSCE	Objective Structured Clinical Examinations
$p(CO_2)$	partial pressure of carbon dioxide
$p(O_2)$	partial pressure of oxygen
PA	posteroanterior
PCA	patient-controlled analgesia
PCOS	polycystic ovary syndrome

PCR	polymerase chain reaction
PE	pulmonary embolus
pg	picogram (i.e. 10^{-12} grams)
PID	pelvic inflammatory disease
PLAB	Professional and Linguistic Assessments Board
POP	progesterone-only pill
prn	*pro re nata* (i.e. as and when needed)
s	second
SaO$_2$	arterial oxygen saturation
sc	subcutaneous
SHO	senior house officer
SOB	shortness of breath
SpO$_2$	oxygen saturation (pulse oximetry)
Staph.	Staphylococcus
STD	sexually transmitted disease
STI	sexually transmitted infection
Strep.	Streptococcus
STRIKES	Setting, paTient's peRception, Invitation, Knowledge, Explore emotions and empathise, Strategy and summary
SVT	supraventricular tachycardia
TB	tuberculosis
TCA	tricyclic antidepressant
TIBC	total iron-binding capacity
U	units
U&E	urea and electrolytes
UTI	urinary tract infection
WBC	white blood count
WCC	white cell count
WPW	Wolff–Parkinson–White (syndrome)

Duties of a doctor

The GMC issues every registered doctor with a number of booklets regarding conduct, etc. The 'Duties of a doctor' comprises a list of 14 principles, and are listed here, word for word, as documented by the GMC.

Patients must be able to trust doctors with their lives and well-being. To justify that trust, we, as a profession, have a duty to maintain a good standard of practice and care and to show respect for human life.

In particular as a doctor you must:
1. Make the care of your patient your first concern.
2. Treat every patient politely and considerately.
3. Respect patients' dignity and privacy.
4. Listen to patients and respect their views.
5. Give patients information in a way they can understand.
6. Respect the rights of patients to be fully involved in decisions about their care.
7. Keep your professional knowledge and skills up to date.
8. Recognise the limits of your professional competence.
9. Be honest and trustworthy.
10. Respect and protect confidential information.
11. Make sure that your personal beliefs do not prejudice your patients' care.
12. Act quickly to protect patients from risk if you have good reason to believe that you or a colleague may not be fit to practise.

13. Avoid abusing your position as a doctor.
14. Work with colleagues in the ways that best serve patients' interests.

In all these matters you must never discriminate unfairly against your patients or colleagues. And you must always be prepared to justify your actions to them.

1

Examinations

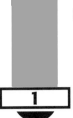

Examination of the systems

Introduction

Systems examinations are your 'bread and butter' for any medical finals exam. However, they have been included here because:

- They appear in the PLAB examination.
- You must shape each examination routine to fit into a 5-minute limit.
- The technique varies slightly from country to country, and you are aiming to adhere to UK set standards.

The following examinations have been included:

- heart and CVS
- respiratory system
- abdomen and GIT
- motor system
- sensory system
- cranial nerves
- peripheral vascular system
- thyroid gland
- breast
- per rectum
- per vagina.

With the obvious exception of the last two examinations, you can practise these on your friends and family until you are confident. Also practise what you would say to the patient as you perform the examination.

2

Examination of the heart and CVS

Please examine the cardiovascular system of this patient.

Answer follows . . .

2

Examination of the heart and CVS

Answer

Examination

Hands

Nails

- Look for splinter haemorrhages, clubbing, peripheral cyanosis.

Palms

- Look for Osler's nodes, Janeway lesions, xanthoma (tendons).

Pulse

- Take the patient's pulse and respiratory rate (mention you would like to have done a radial-radial pulse, a radial-femoral pulse) and check for a collapsing pulse using the brachial artery.

Face

- Look for xanthelasma, any malar flush (mitral stenosis), any central cyanosis.

Mouth

Look inside the mouth for a high-arched palate (Marfan's syndrome). Look at the dentition (infective endocarditis).

Neck

- Look for the jugular venous pulse (JVP) and any other

signs, e.g. Corrigan's pulse.

Chest
Inspection
- Look for any scars around the midline (e.g. coronary artery bypass graft), or left side (mitral valvulotomy).
- Look for any visible pulsations.
- Look at the legs simultaneously for any scars (donor vein grafts), also look for oedema.

Palpation
- Localise the apex beat, can you determine its nature?
- Palpate for a sternal heave.
- Palpate for any P2 pulsation.

Percussion
- The heart borders are generally not percussed.

Auscultation
- Ask the patient to lie in the left lateral position; listen to the mitral area, noting any radiation of murmur to the axilla (found in mitral regurgitation).
- Proceed to auscultate the tricuspid, pulmonary and aortic areas with the patient in the supine position.
- Ask the patient to sit up, breathe out and then in and to hold the breath in inspiration whilst you auscultate the tricuspid and pulmonary areas.
- Now ask the patient to sit up, take a breath in, breathe out and then hold the breath in expiration whilst you auscultate for the aortic area specifically.
- Auscultate the carotids for any bruit or radiation of an ejection systolic murmur (found in aortic stenosis).

Back
Move to the back of the patient.
- Palpate for sacral oedema.

- Percuss for any dullness (effusion).
- Auscultate for any crepitations.

Abdomen
- Palpate for (pulsatile) hepatomegaly.

Legs
- Check if the oedema is pitting.
- Once your examination is complete ask for measurement of:
  - blood pressure
  - peripheral pulses
  - dipstick urine.

Discussion

Be familiar with the various murmurs and the underlying medical conditions. You may be shown an ECG and asked to interpret it.

The different areas of the heart are:
- mitral/apex: left fifth intercostal space, mid-clavicular line
- tricuspid: left sternal edge, fourth intercostal space
- pulmonary: left sternal edge, second intercostal space
- aortic: right sternal edge, second intercostal space.

Holding the breath in inspiration increases venous return to the heart, therefore accentuating any murmurs in the right side of the heart. The reverse is true for murmurs in the left side of the heart.

3

Examination of the respiratory system

A 51-year-old woman, Mrs Khan, is complaining of cough, haemoptysis and breathlessness. Examine her respiratory system and give your diagnosis.

Answer follows . . .

Examination of the respiratory system

Answer

Be aware of the wording in this question. 'Respiratory system' means the whole system; 'Examine this lady's chest' would mean purely focusing on her chest.

Also be aware that 'Khan' is an Asian name and the possibility of TB is always present. However, her age group also makes her a candidate for carcinoma.

Examination

Hands

- Starting with the hands, look for any evidence of:
  - clubbing
  - peripheral cyanosis
  - nicotine staining
  - peripheral wasting
  - flapping tremor.
- Also check her pulse and count her respiratory rate.

Eyes

- Look for Horner's syndrome, jaundice or anaemia.

Face

- Look for any evidence of central cyanosis or pursed-lip breathing.

Neck

- Palpate for any deviation of the trachea.
- Palpate the cricosternal distance using three fingers to rule out tracheal tug (normal distance = 5 cm).
- Palpate for any cervical lymphadenopathy (you should stand behind the patient to do this).
- Look for the jugular venous pulse (JVP).

Chest

Inspection

- Look at the shape of the chest.
- Look for any scars (especially in the back/axilla region).
- Look for any abnormal chest movements.

Palpation, percussion and auscultation

These components are examined anteriorly and posteriorly.

Anteriorly

- Palpation:
  - supraclavicular, supra- and sub-mammary (check for chest expansion)
  - tactile fremitus in the same regions.
- Percussion:
  - supramammary, sub-mammary and axillae (ask the patient to raise her arms).
- Auscultation:
  - supramammary, sub-mammary and axillae
  - check vocal resonance.

Posteriorly

- Ask the patient to fold her arms across her chest and repeat your palpation, percussion and auscultation in the supra- and sub-scapula regions.
- At the end of your examination mention to the examiner that you would:
  - look at the sputum pot

- record the patient's temperature
- note the patient's peak expiratory flow rate.

Discussion

This may seem too much to do within a 5-minute limit; however, you should aim to spend no more than a minute on the first part of the examination. The majority of the time should be spent on examining the chest for findings. You will need to practise this repeatedly so that the procedure looks smooth and professional, and you'll find you **can** do this within the set time.

Possible questions may be related to a chest X-ray present in the cubicle (see the exercise on chest X-ray), peak flow and spirometry (see Chapter 5) and general medical questions related to your diagnosis.

4

Examination of the abdomen and gastrointestinal system

You may be asked, for example, to:

Take a short history and then examine the abdomen of this patient

or

Please examine this patient's gastrointestinal system.

Answer follows . . .

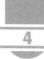

4

Examination of the abdomen and gastrointestinal system

Answer

Always introduce yourself to the patient and obtain their permission to proceed.

In response to the first question take a very short history and then proceed to check the patient and **only** examine the abdomen. To answer the second question conduct a **full** examination as described below.

Examination

Hands
Look for:

- koilonychia – iron deficiency
- leuconychia – cirrhosis
- clubbing – cirrhosis, inflammatory bowel disease
- palmar erythema – cirrhosis
- Dupuytren's contracture – cirrhosis
- pulse – increased in infection, inflammation or bleeding
- flapping tremor/asterixis – cirrhosis or renal failure.

Arms
Look for any:

- scratch marks (pruritus) – liver or renal failure
- needle tracks – intravenous drug abuse (IVDA).

Face
Look for:

- icterus
- pallor
- xanthelasma
- dentition
- angular stomatitis
- glossitis.

Neck

- Make a note to look for Troisier's sign or Virchow's node (an enlarged left-sided supraclavicular lymph node).

Chest

- Look for gynaecomastia or spider naevi.
- Note if the chest hair or axillary hair look diminished.

Abdomen

- Ideally, the patient should be exposed from their nipples to their knees, but it may be impossible to do so during the exam. Exposing the patient down to their pubic hair is probably adequate.

Inspection

- Are the quadrants moving equally?
- Are there any obvious scars or pulsations (bend to the level of the patient's abdomen)?
- Is the umbilicus inverted or everted?
- Is the abdomen flat or distended?
- Are there any obvious masses?

Palpation

- Using the flat of your hand, palpate as the patient inspires.

- Specifically ask the patient about any pain and start palpating from the opposite point of the pain, otherwise palpate from the right iliac fossa, proceeding in a clockwise fashion.
- Palpate the whole abdomen twice: first use gentle palpation to elicit any tenderness, then deeper palpation to look for masses.
- Check for any local rise in temperature. Identify any tender spots.
- Is the abdomen soft, or is there any guarding or rebound?
- Examine for hepatomegaly, starting from the right iliac fossa and working upwards to the right costal margin. Feel for a liver edge moving downwards on respiration.
- Examine for splenomegaly, working from the right iliac fossa to the left costal margin..
- Examine for any abdominal pulsation, check for an expansile impulse in the midline (aortic aneurysm).
- Attempt to ballot each kidney – place the flat of one hand under the patient's loin and use the flat of the fingers of the other hand to feel downwards for a mass in the patient's flank.

Percussion
- Percussion is useful for determining the presence of fluid in the abdomen.
- Percuss from the midline laterally to each flank to check for the presence of fluid. If there is dullness in the flank, ask the patient to lie on one side and percuss again. If the dullness has shifted, this indicates ascites.
- Percuss for a full bladder (suprapubic dullness).
- A very resonant and distended abdomen may suggest bowel obstruction.
- Percussion can also be used to confirm liver span in hepatomegaly – percuss downwards from the right chest anteriorly, starting around the level of the nipple.

- You can generally percuss the abdomen **once** assessing resonance. However, do not needlessly percuss all areas unless you have found an indication to do so.

Auscultation
- Listen for bowel sounds, a normal rate is about 9/min. You are listening specifically for absent or tinkling bowel sounds in the case of bowel obstruction.
- Strictly speaking, 'absent bowel sounds' is defined as no sounds heard during a 3-min period, but the examiner will not expect you to listen for more than approximately 20–30 s.
- Know to check for any bruit over the renal angles.
- Once your examination is completed, say: 'I would like to complete my examination of this patient by examining the hernial orifices and external genitalia, performing a rectal examination and testing the urine'.

Discussion

- The abdomen is a 'Pandora's box' and unfortunately the discussion may lead anywhere!
- Common topics may be liver failure and peripheral signs, and the causes of hepatosplenomegaly.

5

Examination of the motor system

This station may be divided into examination of either the upper or lower limbs.

Neurology examinations are usually feared by candidates because so much is involved. The trick is to keep the following basic examination headings clearly in your mind, and to work through them systematically:
- inspection (attitude, wasting, involuntary movements)
- tone
- power
- reflexes
- gait (in lower limbs).

Examination
- Introduce yourself to the patient and obtain his/her permission to proceed.

Inspection
- Look at the way the limb is held, i.e. its 'attitude', this can give you clues to the diagnosis.
- Look for any wasting of muscle groups.
- Observe for any involuntary movements, which may include fasciculations, tremors, athetosis, etc.

Tone
- Ask the patient if pain is present in any limb before you begin your examination.
- Ask the patient to relax.

- Assess tone by lifting the patient's leg clear off the bed and allowing it to fall back down. In the upper limbs, bend and straighten the limb at the elbow and assess ease of movement.
- Watch for spasticity or rigidity (hypertonia), or flaccidity (hypotonia).

Power
Grade power using the Medical Research Council Grading system:

0 no movement
1 flicker of movement
2 movement without force of gravity (gravity eliminated)
3 movement against force of gravity
4 movement with some added resistance, but not normal
5 movement with full added resistance, normal power.

Ideally, power should be assessed at every joint (adduction, abduction, flexion, extension – as appropriate); however, for a 5-minute OSCE, this may be impossible. Practise fitting in as many as you can in the time:

Shoulder: abduction C4, adduction C5
Elbow: flexion C6, extension C7
Wrist: flexion, extension
Hip: adduction L1–3, abduction L3, flexion L3–4, extension L4–5
Knee: flexion L4–5, extension L3–4
Ankle: dorsiflexion L5, plantar flexion S1

Reflexes
Biceps: C5, C6
Knee: L3, L4
Triceps: C6, C7, C8
Ankle: L5, S1, S2
Supinator: C6
Plantar reflex: S1

Gait

Ask the patient to walk away from the examination couch and back again.

Types of gait

Look for:

- normal gait
- high-stepping gait, slow with careful assessment of movement – peripheral neuropathy
- shuffling gait, small steps, leaning forwards – Parkinson's disease
- circumduction gait, swinging leg around – hemiplegia
- wide-based gait – cerebellar disease or sensory ataxia (dorsal column dysfunction).

Discussion

Correct positioning of the patient while testing for reflexes is all-important. A little practise goes a long way to making this part of the examination look confident and slick.

Biceps: Place your thumb over the biceps tendon and strike the tendon hammer over this tendon. Watch for contraction of the biceps muscle.

Triceps: Allow the patient to relax their arm on yours, isolate the triceps tendon and strike the tendon hammer directly onto it. Watch for contraction of the triceps muscle.

Supinator: Find and strike the tendon to the brachioradialis (lateral aspect of the forearm just proximal to the wrist). Watch for flexion and supination of the forearm.

Knee: Ask the patient to flex their knees (to about 30°), place your arm under the patient's knees and take their weight on it. Isolate the patella tendon and strike it with the tendon hammer. Watch for extension of the knee and contraction of the quadriceps muscle.

Ankle: Instruct the patient to externally rotate the leg, flex it at the knee and dorsiflex at the ankle. Stabilise the Achilles tendon by holding the forefoot and strike the Achilles tendon. Watch for plantar flexion and contraction in the calf muscles.

Plantar: This is uncomfortable, warn the patient first. Run a key or orange-stick along the lateral border of the foot from the heel upwards. You may need to hold the ankle to avoid a withdrawal reflex. Watch the toes for fanning and extension (positive Babinski sign). **Never** use the sharp end of the tendon hammer as this is rarely clean and may be too sharp – examiners will frown at anyone who does this!

6

Examination of the sensory system

Here, you could be asked to examine either the upper or lower limbs of a person. There may be clues in the question, for example indicating that the patient is diabetic or is known to abuse alcohol. The headings to include in your examination are:

- pain
- temperature
- light touch
- joint position sense
- vibration
- co-ordination.

Examination

Pain and temperature

Both pain and temperature sensations are carried through the lateral spinothalamic tract.

Pain

Assessing for pain is an important part of the sensory examination, but be careful **not to hurt the patient**. Using a sterile pin, do a check test (usually over the patient's sternum) to ensure the patient is able to perceive the 'sharp' sensation. Then proceed to test the dermatomes over the relevant limbs (upper or lower).

Light touch

The above test for pain should be repeated using a cotton wisp to assess light touch.

Temperature

Usually, a test for temperature involves holding test tubes filled with hot and cold water against the patient's skin and asking them to differentiate hot from cold. Although this test is rarely used, the candidate should be aware of it.

Joint position sense

Joint position sense is carried through the posterior dorsal columns.

- Holding the sides of the patient's finger or toe, demonstrate up and down movements, notifying the patient which movement is up and which is down.
- Ask the patient to close their eyes, then repeat the up or down manoeuvre asking the patient to specify the direction of movement.

Vibration

Vibration, like joint position sense is carried through the posterior columns.

The standard method for testing vibration sense in the periphery employs a 128-Hz tuning fork. (This is a good test for peripheral neuropathy, e.g. alcohol abuse/diabetes.)

- Place the vibrating tuning fork on a bony prominence (the sternum may be used as a control) and ask the patient to indicate when the vibration stops.
- Then repeat with the patient's eyes closed, starting at the most distal bony prominence (e.g. the first metatarsophalangeal joint in the lower limbs). If the vibration sense is impaired, move one joint proximally.

Co-ordination

There are several tests for co-ordination, which primarily reflect cerebellar activity:

- **Upper limbs** – you could ask the patient to touch your finger and then their own nose, repeatedly and as fast as possible; note for past pointing, intention tremor and their speed of response.

- **Lower limbs** – here, the heel-to-shin test is commonly used. The patient lies down and is asked to place the heel of one foot onto the knee of their other leg, and then slide it straight down the shin. Repeat on the other side.

Romberg's test
Ask the patient to stand with their feet together. Look for any postural imbalance. Conduct the test with the patient's eyes open, and then with their eyes closed.
- If sway is noted with their eyes closed – this is due to a lack of sensory proprioception (sensory ataxia). This is a positive test.
- If sway is noted with their eyes open or closed – this indicates cerebellar disease (cerebellar ataxia). This is **not** a positive test.

Discussion

Distribution of the dermatomes
(A rough guide only, reference to precise anatomical models is recommended)

Upper limbs
C5 – radial side arm
C6 – radial side forearm
C7 – middle finger to forearm
C8 – ulnar side hand
T1 – ulnar side forearm
T2 – medial side arm

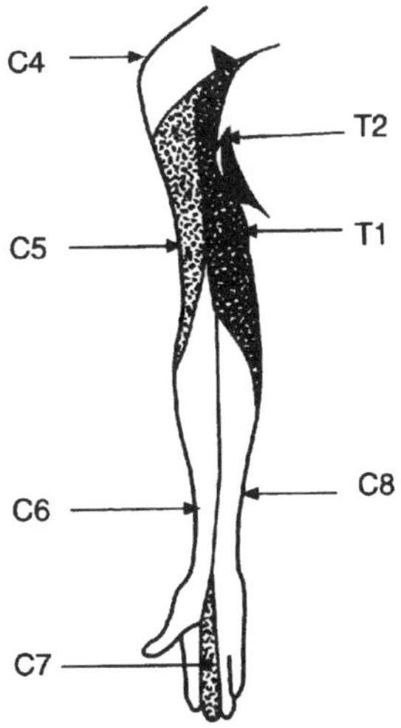

Figure 1.1 Upper limb dermatones.

Lower limbs

L1 – ilioinguinal region
L2 – front of the thigh
L3 – over the knee
L4 – medial aspect of the lower leg
L5 – lateral aspect of the lower leg*
S1 – lateral border of the foot/plantar aspect

(*Note that L5 also supplies a small patch between the first and second toes.)

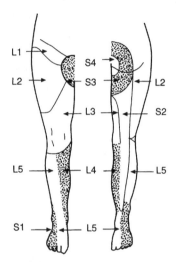

Figure 1.2 Lower limb dermatones.

Cerebellar signs
Look for:

- nystagmus
- hypotonia
- intension tremor
- rebound phenomenon
- dysdiadochokinesia
- slow scanning speech.

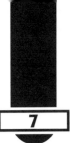

7

Examination of the cranial nerves

Ms Ganglion is a 37-year-old woman who has experienced a sudden onset of left-sided facial weakness, she denies any hearing loss or skin vesicles. Please examine Ms Ganglion's cranial nerves.

Answer follows . . .

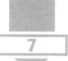

7

Examination of the cranial nerves

Answer

The cranial nerve station is usually divided into two halves – you will either be asked to examine cranial nerves II–VII or VII–XII. As with all the stations it takes practice. However, once mastered it is easy to complete this station well within the allocated time, and to make it look very smooth.

Examination

Introduce yourself to the patient and obtain her permission to proceed.

Cranial nerve I

This is the olfactory nerve and, generally, is not examined in this station. If, however, it is included then you can ask the patient about any recent change in her ability to smell. (Classically, smell is tested by blindfolding the patient and asking them to identify common aromatic agents, such as coffee. Irritants such as ammonia should **not** be used.)

Cranial nerves II–VII

Cranial nerves II, III, IV, VI (the optic, oculomotor, trochlear and abducens nerves)

These comprise many components, including: colour vision, visual acuity, eye movements, accommodation

reflex, light reflex (direct and indirect), visual fields, and
fundoscopy.

It may be impossible to cover all the components in great
detail within the time limit, but the essential points for the
PLAB exam are given below.

- **Colour vision**: Ask the patient if they wear glasses, ask
  them to identify primary colours such as red and green
  (colour vision).
- **Visual acuity**: If they wear glasses, ask the patient to put
  them on and test visual acuity by asking the patient to
  read the top line of a newspaper, or by finger counting.
- **Visual field assessment**: Sit directly opposite the patient
  and, using the confrontation method, assess the four
  quadrants, identifying any blind spots that do not
  correlate with your own (assuming you have normal
  fields).
- **Accommodation reflex**: Finally move your finger closer
  to the patient (moving your finger towards the top of
  their nose) and watch their eyes for the accommodation
  reflex as you get closer to a point between their eyes.
- **Eye movements**: Test by using your finger as a focus
  point and drawing a giant letter 'H' in the air, always
  watching the patient's eyes throughout the horizontal
  and vertical components of movement (up, down, left
  and right). When at the right or left of the field, ask the
  patient to hold their focus and keep your finger still for a
  few seconds, assess for the presence of any nystagmus.
  Ask the patient if he/she is experiencing any diplopia
  (double vision). Be careful not to get the patient to look
  too far to either side as this causes nystagmus in normal
  subjects – try it!

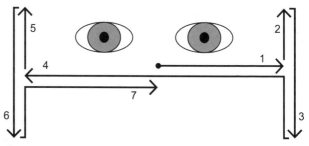

Figure 1.3

- **Light reflex**: Using a pen torch, look for the direct and indirect pupillary reflexes. Shine the light into each eye **twice**.
- **Fundoscopy**: Mention that if time permitted you would like to conduct a fundoscopic examination (described in Chapter 5).

Cranial nerve V (the trigeminal nerve)
Remember this nerve has both sensory and motor functions.
- Check sensation bilaterally in divisions V1 (ophthalmic), V2 (maxillary) and V3 (mandibular) on the forehead, cheek and chin.
- Test the motor component by asking the patient to clench their teeth, then feel for clenching of the masseters and temporalis on each side.
- Assess the action of the pterygoids by asking the patient to move their lower jaw from side to side.
- Look for any symmetry in the creases of the nasolabial folds.

Cranial nerve VII (the facial nerve)
- Ask the patient to keep their head still and look upwards, note any wrinkle formation across the forehead.
- Ask the patient to squeeze their eyes tight shut as you try to force them open.

- Ask the patient to smile, preferably showing their teeth. Look for any facial droop.

Cranial nerves VII–XII (the facial, vestibulocochlear, glossopharyngeal, vagus, spinal accessory, hypoglossal nerves)

Cranial VII nerve (the facial nerve)
See above.

Cranial VIII nerve (the vestibulocochlear nerve)
Assessment of this nerve classically includes testing for hearing, using the Rinne and Weber's tests. Balance can also be assessed.

However for the PLAB examination, simply acknowledge the presence of this nerve by testing the patient's hearing. Close the tragus of the opposite ear and whisper a number into the patient's ear, ask the patient to repeat the number out loud. Repeat on the opposite side.

IX–X nerves (the glossopharyngeal and vagus nerves)
Ask the patient to say 'aahh' loudly and look for a centrally placed uvula and symmetrical movements of the soft palate. Rule out muscle fatigue (myasthenia gravis) by requesting the patient to repeat 'la, la, la, la, la' for a few seconds.

XI nerve (the spinal accessory nerve)
Ask the patient to shrug both shoulders as you try to oppose this action, brought about by the trapezius muscle. Ask the patient to push your hand away using the side of their face, look for the contraction of the sternomastoid on the opposite side.

XII nerve (the hypoglossal nerve)
Assess for any fasciculations while the tongue is relaxed in

the mouth. Ask the patient to stick out their tongue, look for any deviation to any side indicating weakness on that particular side.

Discussion

- **Olfactory nerve:** The commonest cause of anosmia is the common cold. Other causes include trauma to the cribriform plate and various syndromes, e.g. Kallman's syndrome.
- **Optic, oculomotor, trochlear and abducens nerves:** It is worth knowing how to recognise a IIIn palsy or a VIn palsy. A IIIn palsy of vascular origin (e.g. hypertension and diabetes) tends to be pupil-sparing.
- **Facial nerve:** A lower motor neurone lesion involves the whole side of the face with loss of forehead wrinkles and a facial droop. An upper motor neurone lesion will involve only the lower quadrant of the face (facial droop only). The frontalis muscle receives bilateral innervation and is therefore spared in a patient with an upper motor nerve lesion. Although it is impractical to attempt to test for, remember that VIIn also has branches to the anterior two-thirds of the tongue and the stapedius (middle ear).
- **Glossopharyngeal and vagus nerves:** Classically, these are tested for by the 'gag reflex'. However, this is no longer considered to be good practice as it causes the patient to retch and is an unreliable sign, being absent in 10% of normal subjects. Instead, you can ask the patient to swallow while you feel for movement of their larynx.

8

Examination of the lower limbs (peripheral vascular system)

Imagine you are an SHO working on an endocrinology firm, you are in the diabetes clinic. Please tell me what things you might want to check in a patient who has come for an annual check-up and then proceed to conduct an examination of the lower limbs.

Answer follows . . .

8

Examination of the lower limbs (peripheral vascular system)

Answer

You need to practise this station and time yourself.

Key points in a diabetic annual check-up

- Introduce yourself to the patient and ask if they are having any particular problems. If so, are these consistent with their medication?
- Check the patient's body weight and compare it with previous records.
- Look at the patient's home blood glucose (capillary blood glucose) records.
- Take blood samples for: glucose, lipids, Hb A_{1C}, U&E.
- Ask for a urine sample for: glucose, ketones and protein.
- Examine the eyes:
  - for xanthelasma, corneal arcus (hypercholesterolaemia)
  - to assess visual acuity (maculopathy)
  - to check eye movements (mononeuritis multiplex affecting cranial nerves III, IV, VI)
  - by fundoscopy, looking for cataract, rubeosis iridis, retinopathy, vitreous haemorrhage.
- Look in the mouth for candidiasis (oral thrush).
- Listen in the neck for a carotid bruit (atherosclerosis).
- Check the blood pressure (should check with the patient lying and standing to test for postural hypotension).
- Examine the chest for any signs of chest infection or

pulmonary oedema.
- Examine insulin injection sites (if relevant) for evidence of lipohypertrophy.

Lower limb examination
Inspection
Feet: ulcers, signs of pre-gangrene, infections between the toes or at any sites of injury, muscle wasting, pes cavus/claw toes
Ankles: Charcot's joints (any deformity)
Leg: muscle wasting
Knee: Charcot's joints
Thigh: injection sites for lipoatrophy, wasting of the quadriceps, diabetic amyotrophy.

Palpation
Pulses: dorsalis pedis (naturally absent in up to 14% of people), posterior tibial, femoral
Reflexes: ankle, knee, plantar (extensor in diabetic amyotrophy)
Sensory examination (testing predominantly for functions of the posterior column):
- *touch* (first test on the sternum so the patient knows what to expect):
  - fine touch: test with a wisp of cotton-wool
  - pain: test with a disposable pin for pinprick sensation
  - deep pain: test with firm pressure over the toenails. If not felt, move up to the calves
- joint-position sense:
  - start at the metatarsophalangeal joints. If absent, move up to the ankles, then the knees
- *vibration sense* (test on the sternum):
  - start at the base of the great toe. If absent, move to medial malleolus, tibial shaft, tibial tuberosity, anterior iliac crest
- temperature:

     ○ warm and cold water to touch (you are unlikely to be asked to do this in the exam.)
- *diabetes mellitus*: note the pattern of sensory loss in such patients:
  - early loss: vibration sense, deep pain, temperature
  - late loss: joint-position sense.

Power (Grade 0–5)

Check movements at the:
- **hip joint**: flexion, extension, abduction, adduction
- **knee joint**: flexion, extension
- **ankle joint**: dorsiflexion and plantar flexion
- **metatarsophalangeal joints** (MTPJs): flexion and extension

Finally

Ask the patient to walk and perform Romberg's test (posterior column disease).

Examination of the thyroid gland (examination of the neck)

This 5-minute station may simply read:

'Examination of the thyroid gland'

or

'Examination of the neck'.

Alternatively, it may say:

'Please adopt the role of an SHO in an endocrinology clinic'.

Answer follows . . .

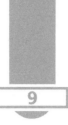

9

Examination of the thyroid gland (examination of the neck)

Answer

Practise talking your way through the examination, exaggerating the steps so the examiner can clearly see what you are looking for. However, do not be surprised if the examiner asks you to stop talking and get on with it! In which case remain silent but show each step clearly, you may be asked questions at the end.

Examination

Introduce yourself to the patient, explain that you need to examine her neck and obtain her permission to proceed.

Hands

- Shake hands with the patient: are their hands cold/sweating; is the skin thickened; are there obvious tremors?
- Look for thyroid acropachy (similar to clubbing).
- Look for onycholysis in the nails.
- Look for palmar erythema.
- Ask the patient to stretch out her arms to look for fine tremor.
- Check the pulse for tachycardia or bradycardia.
- Look for proximal myopathy.

Face

Patients with myxoedema often have a characteristic

'peaches and cream' complexion. They may also have dry skin and hair.

- Note any obvious loss of hair (alopecia) or thinning.
- Look for eye signs: exophthalmos, lid lag, ophthalmoplegia, lid retraction, absence of forehead wrinkling.

Neck

Inspection

- Is there any obvious mass? Look at the front and sides of the neck.
- Decide whether this is a thyroid mass or if it could be lymphadenopathy.
- Ask the patient to take a sip of water – an enlarged thyroid gland or thyroglossal cyst will rise on swallowing, this is due to an attachment to the larynx via the ligament of Berry.
- Ask the patient to stick out her tongue – only a thyroglossal cyst will rise on protrusion.

Palpation

- Standing behind the patient (tell the patient what you are going to do) use the fingertips of both your hands to feel for the lobes and isthmus.
- Assess for size, shape and consistency. Feel for a lower border (upon swallowing) and always ask about tenderness.
- Examine for cervical lymphadenopathy.
- Feel for the position of the trachea.

Percussion

- Percuss over the suprasternal notch to rule out a retrosternal thyroid.

Auscultation

- A bruit may be present due to increased vascularity. Be

careful to listen over the goitre and not the carotid arteries.

Discussion

- Time permitting, what other examinations might you want to conduct?:
  - examination of the lower limbs for reflexes at the knee and ankle
  - inspection for pre-tibial myxoedema (a sign of hyperthyroidism – specific to Grave's disease).
- What investigations would you request?

10

Examination of the breast

Ms Reynolds, a 19-year-old woman, has presented at her GP surgery anxious that her breast feels 'lumpy' and unsure if this is abnormal for her. She has a family history of breast cancer, including her maternal aunt and grandmother.

Answer follows . . .

10

Examination of the breast

Answer

A manikin will be present for this station. Because it may incorporate various features, you should be familiar with basic management procedures and initial investigations. However, this station is predominantly an assessment of your examination skills, and therefore it is important that you know how to conduct such an examination correctly. **Remember** not to talk to the manikin.

Examination

- Mention that you would introduce yourself to the patient.
- Explain that you need to examine the patient's breasts and that you would obtain the patient's permission to proceed.
- Say that you would ask the patient to undress to the waist.
- Tell the examiner you would ensure the patient's privacy and the presence of a chaperone.

Inspection

This is performed with the patient in the following four positions: arms by the sides; arms raised above the head; hands pressing onto the hips; bending over.

Look for any:
- asymmetry, and at the size, shape and contours of the breasts

- puckering or discoloration of the skin, peau d'orange and nodules
- inversion/retraction, any obvious discharge, displacement or deviation of the nipples
- cracks in the areola, enlarged tubercles and change in colour
- swelling (lymphoedema) of the arms.

Palpation

This is best conducted with the patient in the 45° recumbent position (on the couch).

Remember to rub your hands together to warm them up before examining the patient.

Examine the patient's breasts using the flat of your fingers, palmar aspect, and examine the normal breast first.
- Note the temperature of the breasts.
- Look for any swelling/lump; if so, describe its size, shape, colour, consistency.
- Note if the swelling is fixed to:
  - the skin (unable to pinch the skin over it)
  - underlying muscles (more prominent on tensing the pectoral muscles).
- Check if the swelling is fixed to one or both planes (attempt to move it vertically and horizontally).
- Tell the examiner you would ask the patient if she has any discharge from a nipple. If so, ask her to express it for you, noting its colour and consistency.
- Palpate for axillary and supraclavicular nodes. If present, describe them by number, size, consistency, and note whether they are tender and fixed. To examine the left axilla, hold the patient's left forearm with your left forearm. use the palmar aspect of the fingers of your right hand to palpate lymph nodes in the axilla – anterior, posterior, medial, lateral and deep (high up in

the axilla). Repeat for the right axilla.
- Mention at the end that you would examine the patient's abdomen for any hepatosplenomegaly/ascites and the spine for any bony tenderness.

Discussion

Types of discharge from the nipple

Colour	Cause
Blood:	duct papilloma
Pink (serum and blood):	duct carcinoma
Clear/pale yellow/pus:	duct ectasia
Brown:	duct ectasia
Green/black:	cysts
Milky/thin:	lactation

First-line investigations
- An ultrasound scan and mammogram should be performed.
- Anything cystic that **does not** seem to be malignant will need fine-needle aspiration (FNA) for cytology. Beyond this, an excision biopsy will be required to determine the nature of the cellular growth.

11

Mini-mental state examination – standardised

There are many variations on the Mini-Mental State Examination, but the one discussed here is the standardised version (adapted from Molloy, D.W., *et al.* (1991). Reliability of a Standardized Mini-Mental State Examination compared with the traditional Mini-Mental State Examination. *American Journal of Psychiatry*, **140**, 102–5.)

You should become familiar with the following set of questions, as there is a lot to ask, often in a short amount of time (about 5 minutes).

Questions

1. (Allow 10 seconds for each reply.)
    o What year is this? (Exact answer only, unless just into a new year.)
    o What season is this? (Can accept previous or after if turn of season.)
    o What month of the year is this? (On first day of new month or last day of previous, accept either.)
    o What date is it? (Accept exact date ± 1 day.)
    o What day of the week is this? (Exact day only.)
    o Score one point for each correct answer.
2. (Allow 10 seconds for each reply.)
    o What country are we in? (Correct answer only.)
    o What county are we in? (Accept a reasonable answer like 'Greater Manchester' instead of 'Lancashire'.)
    o What city/town are we in? (Correct answer only.)

- (In clinic): What is the name of this hospital/building? (Correct answer only.)
- (In home): What is the street address of this house? (Street and number.)
- (In clinic): What floor of the building are we on? (Correct answer only.)
- (In home): What room are we in? (Correct answer only.)
- Score one point for each correct answer.

3. I am going to name three objects. After I have said all three, I want you to repeat them. Remember them, as I am going to ask you what they were in a few minutes time. (Say them slowly at approximately 1-second intervals):

- ball (example of alternatives: bell, bull)
- car (jar, tar)
- man (fan, pan)

Please repeat the three objects.

Score one point for each correct repetition on the first attempt, allow 20 seconds for reply. If all 3 not repeated, repeat until they are learned up to a maximum of five times before moving on.

4. Spell the word 'WORLD' (you may help them.) Now ask them to spell it backwards. Allow 30 seconds. Maximum score 5, minus 1 mark for each mistake. Score 0 if they cannot spell 'WORLD' even with assistance.

5. What were the three objects I asked you to remember? Allow 10 seconds. 1 point for each correct response regardless of order.

6. Show the patient a wristwatch, ask them to name it. 1 point for the correct answer. Do not accept 'time', 'clock', etc.

7. Show a pen. Ask them to name it. 1 point for the correct answer. Do not accept 'pencil'.

8. Repeat after me: 'No ifs, ands, or buts'. Exact phrase only scores 1 point.

9. 'Read the words on this page and do what it says.' Hand

the patient a sheet with the order 'CLOSE YOUR EYES' on it. Score 1 point for the correct response, allowing 10 seconds. Subject must close their eyes, but does not have to read aloud. You can repeat the instructions up to 3 times.

10. Ask the patient if they are left-/right-handed. Hold a piece of paper in front of them and ask them to:

  o take it in their non-dominant hand
  o fold it in half
  o put it on the floor.

Allow 30 seconds. Score 1 point for each correct action (maximum of three).

11. Give the subject something to write with, and a piece of paper. Ask them to write any complete sentence. The sentence must be grammatically correct, but ignore spelling errors. Score one point for correct response.

12. Place a design (see Figure 1.4), pencil, eraser and paper in front of the subject. Ask them to copy it. Allow multiple tries until they hand it back. Score 1 point if correct. There must be a four-sided figure between the two pentagons. Allow 1 minute.

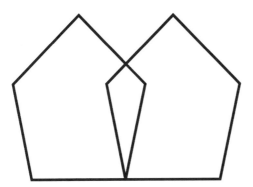

Figure 1.4

Discussion

A score of 24/30 or better is normal. Serial examination scores may be required to obtain a more accurate guide to the patient's state. **Remember** the examination is not a diagnosis by itself, but rather a screening test for cognitive impairment.

2

History taking

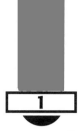

1

Asthma

You are the SHO in A&E when Mr Jones, a 23-year-old man, is brought in suffering an acute asthma attack. Please take a history from this patient.

Answer follows . . .

Asthma

Answer

Asthma is a chronic and common problem. When an asthmatic patient presents to you, it is usually a case of some urgency.

The emergency management of acute asthma is dealt with in Chapter 6. However, it is important for the PLAB exam (and for all practical purposes) to keep a framework of questions ingrained in your mind, so when the situation arises you will be able to deal with it quickly and effectively.

Rather than providing a simulated conversation, this section gives a list of relevant history-taking questions, followed by a discussion of the salient points.

Questions to ask the patient

Presenting complaint

- How long have suffered with asthma? (years)
- Is it usually well controlled?
- When did you start becoming short of breath? (over days/hours)
- When do you normally become short of breath? (early morning/evening/weekends)
- How many times in a day/night do you use your blue inhaler (reliever)?
- What is your best peak flow reading? (L/min)
- What is your best exercise tolerance? (metres/yards)

Exacerbating factors
- Have you recently had a cough/produced sputum?
- Have you recently moved house/started a new job/had any upsets?
- Do you have any pets?
- Are you allergic to house dust or anything else?
- Have you started any new exercises or habits (smoking)?

Past history
- Have you ever been hospitalised for your asthma?
- Have you ever needed to be put onto a ventilator to help you breathe? (ITU admission)
- Do you have eczema or hayfever/any other medical conditions?

Family history
- Does anybody else in your family suffer with asthma/eczema? (atopy)

Drug history
- Are you allergic to any drugs?
- What medication(s) do you take for asthma?
- Do you take your medicine regularly?
- Do you have a home nebuliser or oxygen?

Note: Check the patient's other medication, both prescribed and those purchased over-the-counter, for possible side-effects (e.g. NSAIDs/beta-blockers).

Social history
- Do you smoke? How many?
- Do you drink? How much?
- What is your occupation?
- Are you suffering a lot of stress at present?

Discussion

Read the related topics in Chapter 5 regarding the correct inhaler technique and use of the peak expiratory flow meter.

Familiarise yourself with the BTS (British Thoracic Society) guidelines for the treatment of asthma, these may be found in the *BNF* (*British National Formulary*).

2

Vaginal bleeds

Imagine you are working in the A&E department as an SHO, a 28-year-old woman comes to you after 8 weeks of amenorrhoea, complaining of vaginal bleeding. Please take a history and state your further management.

Answer follows . . .

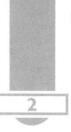

2

Vaginal bleeds

Answer

This is a fairly typical PLAB question. Following some important basic principles will help you to reach a diagnosis and formulate your management plans for any woman with an abnormal vaginal bleed.

Key points

- Is the woman of reproductive age or post-menopausal?
- If she is of reproductive age, is she pregnant or not?
- If she is pregnant, is she less than 20 weeks' or more than 20 weeks' gestation?

Rule 1: All women of childbearing age are assumed to be pregnant until proven otherwise.

Post-menopausal bleeding is generally not something that can be dealt with in an A&E department, and so the patient needs to be referred to the gynaecology department. Some causes may include carcinoma of the cervix, endometrium, etc.

A non-pregnant woman presenting with a vaginal bleed (unless trauma has been involved, or the bleeding is torrential), is again not something that should be dealt with in an A&E department, she can be given advice and sent for follow-up with her GP or a specialist. Causes can include pelvic inflammatory disease (PID), fibroids, cervical erosion, etc.

A pregnant woman of more than 20 weeks' gestation presenting with an abnormal vaginal bleed could have a placenta praevia or a placenta abruptio, and ideally needs fast-track referral to obstetrics for specialist management on admission.

If the pregnancy is less than 20 weeks' gestation you could be looking at an ectopic pregnancy, a miscarriage/abortion, or an abnormal conception (e.g. molar pregnancy). Each of these should be identified and dealt with appropriately.

Rule 2: All pregnancies should be assumed to be ectopic until proven otherwise.

Key points in an ectopic pregnancy (significant pain, scanty bleeding)

- Classically, an ectopic pregnancy presents after 6–8 weeks' amenorrhoea.
- The bleeding is darker red/brown and scanty (spotting).
- There is significant abdominal pain (noticed before the vaginal spotting).
- There may be a history of using an IUCD (this can increase the chance of an ectopic pregnancy).
- An adnexal mass may be palpable on pelvic examination.
- A ruptured ectopic pregnancy can result in collapse and shock.

Key points in a miscarriage/abortion (profuse bleeding, less pain)

- The different types of abortion include: 'threatened', 'inevitable', 'complete'.
- In threatened abortion the woman feels all the symptoms but the embryo is intact. This can further progress to an inevitable abortion where the conception products are expelled with bleeding and pain. When the pain and bleeding has subsided the cervical os closes and the process is complete.

- The bleeding here tends to be heavy and bright red, fresh blood with 'clots' (i.e. possible products of conception).
- The pain may be noticed after the onset of bleeding.

Questions to ask the patient

General

- When did the bleeding start?
- Which came first, the bleeding or the pain?
- Is the bleeding heavy with clots or slight?
- Is it fresh, bright-red blood or a darkish colour?
- Describe the pain (site, onset, character, radiation, severity, associated features, any aggravating/relieving factors)?
- Have you had a previous ectopic pregnancy, how does the pain compare this time?
- Is there any chance you may be pregnant? (Any changes such as morning sickness, breast tenderness and enlargement?)
- Have you noticed any dysuria?
- Do you open your bowels regularly/is everything normal?
- Have you any bleeding from other sites?
- How are you in yourself? Have you experienced any stress/lifted anything heavy recently, etc.

Menstrual history

- What was the date of your last menstrual period?
- Are your periods usually regular? What's the duration? (e.g. 4/28-day cycles)
- Do you have any pain/problems with your periods?

Obstetric history

If possible, calculate the parity index; if not, just ask about any previous pregnancy.

- When was your last pregnancy?

- Was it a normal delivery at term?
- Did you have a Caesarean section, was it elective or an emergency?
- Did you have an assisted delivery, what was the indication for it?

Past medical history

- Do you have any other medical problems? (particularly haematological/bleeding disorders)

Drug history

- Are you on any medication? (particularly aspirin or anticoagulants)
- Do you use any form of contraception? (Ensure the patient is fully compliant.)

Management plan

Rule 3: Ensure a chaperone is present!

1. Conduct a general systems' examination. You may conduct a pelvic examination. if you feel you are capable, if not save time and leave this for the specialist. However, you may want to be familiar with the findings in case you are asked (documented above).
2. Perform a pregnancy test.
3. If you suspect an ectopic pregnancy or an abortion (or just a very heavy vaginal bleed) insert a wide-bore cannula.
4. Take blood samples for a full blood count, a Group and Save Serum (GSS) (cross-match if urgent), ABO group and rhesus typing.
5. Baseline serum βHCG is helpful in correlating with the duration of pregnancy. Normally it increases by 60% or above every 48 hours. Any deviation from this should be treated with suspicion of abnormal pregnancy, irrespective of its site. It is important to do a baseline

serum βHCG when you see a patient with suspected ectopic pregnancy in A&E.

6. Discuss the case with the on-call SHO in obstetrics/gynaecology. Most likely the patient will be admitted and booked in for an ultrasound scan. The patient should be kept nil by mouth.

Subsequent management of an ectopic pregnancy includes serial im injections of methotrexate, and possibly salpingotomy or salpingectomy. This may require the patient to stay in hospital for up to 2–5 days, and to rest at home for 4 weeks.

An abortion or miscarriage is usually allowed to progress naturally, with resuscitative measures for the mother.

3

Vaginal discharge

A 20-year-old woman presents to you in the clinic complaining of dyspareunia and a foul-smelling PV discharge. Take a history and outline your management.

This question can be used to cover history taking for both PID and sexually transmitted diseases (STDs). As the two topics are quite interlinked, we will deal with them both here rather than separately.

PID, or pelvic inflammatory disease, as the name suggests, is inflammation of the female reproductive organs secondary to infection. This infection may or may not be sexually transmitted.

Pelvic inflammatory disease

History

The patient (usually a young adult) generally gives a history of lower abdominal pain, which is normally constant and dragging in nature. Start by asking the patient about her symptoms. Apart from lower abdominal pain, patients may also give a history of painful intercourse or dyspareunia. Sometimes they also complain of menstrual irregularities, e.g. intermenstrual bleeding, post-coital bleeding or menorrhagia. They may also report painful micturation or dysuria. Vaginal discharge may or may not be present:

- A greenish discharge is usually secondary to infection with *Pseudomonas* spp.
- A fishy-smelling discharge is due to *Trichomonas vaginalis.*
- A white, curdy discharge is due to *Candida albicans* or

thrush.
- Sometimes you can also have excessive leucorrhoea or a white vaginal discharge without an infection.

You should also ask about a recent termination of pregnancy. The incidence of post-abortion PID is high and secondary infertility is one of the sequels of PID.

Diagnosis
This is usually clinched by finding pelvic tenderness or a mass on bimanual examination and cervical excitation.

Investigations
- A FBC should be performed and CRP (C-reactive protein) measured.
- Urethral, high-vaginal and endocervical swabs should be taken to look for *Chlamydia* and *Gonococcus* spp.
- A mid-stream urine sample should be sent for culture and sensitivity testing.

Treatment

If you clinically suspect PID then you should start treatment empirically, without waiting for the swabs to come back as positive. The most recommended treatment is the triple antibiotic regimen of 100 mg doxycycline twice daily for 7 days, along with 400 mg metronidazole three times a day and 500 mg cefalexin three times a day for 5 days.

Sexually transmitted diseases
History
If you are given the same scenario and asked to take a history for sexually transmitted disease then, apart from asking the same questions regarding symptoms, you also need to take a detailed sexual history. You need to know

whether the patient is in a stable relationship with a single partner. It is sometimes a difficult situation when, although the patient is being faithful, the partner may be unfaithful. You also have to know whether the patient is in a heterosexual, homosexual or bisexual relationship. This will give you an idea of the kind of infections to expect. It is very important to know what kind of contraceptive the couple is using: condoms are the most effective contraceptive in preventing STDs. You also have to know whether the patient uses illicit drugs; studies have shown that drug users are more prone to contracting STDs.

Investigations and treatment

The investigations for sexually transmitted disease are the same as for PID. However, if the patient is screened positive for any STD then she and her partner(s) are referred to the GUM (genitourinary medicine) clinic. This is not only essential for treatment, but is also very important for contact tracing to prevent further spread of the disease.

4

Amenorrhoea

Mrs Cunningham, a 36-year-old woman presents with amenorrhoea of 9 months' duration. Please take a history from her and present your differential diagnosis.

Answer follows . . .

4

Amenorrhoea

Answer

Now unless you are a gynaecology specialist, this question needs some thinking about because there are more causes for amenorrhoea than simple pregnancy! (**Remember Rule 1.**) Any woman presenting with amenorrhoea is pregnant till proven otherwise. Pregnancy testing is essential. It is better to understand the causes of the patient's amenorrhoea rather than trying to memorise a list from an answer given in a book. This question refers to secondary amenorrhoea (i.e. because Mrs Cunningham was menstruating until 9 months ago).

By going back to basics and understanding the mechanisms behind the onset of secondary amenorrhoea, you can elicit a history based on the physiology. The basic mechanism underlying menstruation involves the HPO axis (hypothalamic-pituitary-ovarian, **remember**!). The hypothalamus stimulates the pituitary to secrete pulsatile gonadotrophins, such as FSH (follicle-stimulating hormone) and LH (luteinising hormone), which in turn stimulate the ovaries to release oestrogen and progesterone. The entire cycle is modulated by feedback from the ovaries to the hypothalamus and the pituitary. Therefore, anything that upsets any one component of this cycle can result in secondary amenorrhoea:

- **HPO axis causes** of secondary amenorrhoea are common, e.g. emotions, stress, weight loss, anorexia nervosa, hyperthyroidism, pituitary tumours (which secrete excess prolactin), Sheehan's syndrome (pituitary necrosis in the post-partum period). The latter two causes are less common.

- **Ovarian causes** include polycystic ovary syndrome, ovarian tumours and primary ovarian failure (i.e. premature menopause).
- **Uterine causes** may be due to Asherman's syndrome (uterine adhesions due to a previous dilatation and curettage procedure) and post-Pill amenorrhoea, which is usually oligomenorrhoea masked by regular withdrawal bleeds whilst on the contraceptive pill.

Keeping the above differential diagnoses in mind, you can now form a framework for taking the patient's history.

Questions to ask the patient

Menstrual history

- How old were you when you had your first period?
- Were your periods regular until 9 months ago? Were they heavy or light? Any pain/problems? How long did they last for?
- When was your last menstrual period (LMP)?

Obstetric history

- Have you conceived in the past? Did it go to term? Was it a normal delivery?
- Did you have any problems in the post-partum period, e.g. any heavy bleeding? (Sheehan's syndrome).
- Have you ever had a pregnancy terminated? Have you ever had a D&C (dilatation and curettage)? (Asherman's syndrome)

Previous medical history

- Have you every suffered with thyroid problems (dislike of warm environments, tremors, sweating/the opposite)?
- Are you overweight? Have you noticed any recent

changes in yourself, such as facial hair or a deepening voice? (polycystic ovaries)

- Have you noticed any discharge from your nipples, or tunnel vision? (pituitary tumour)
- Have you noticed your stomach increasing in size, or can you feel a swelling in your tummy? (ovarian tumour)
- How are you in yourself? Have you had a cough or fever? Do you feel tired or unwell? (systemic illness)
- Are you eating and drinking well? Have you lost any weight recently? (anorexia/bulimia)

Drug history

- Are you on any prescribed/over-the-counter/herbal medication? (drug side-effects)
- Do you use or have you used the Pill? (post-pill amenorrhoea)

Family history

- When did your mother/sisters reach the menopause? (perimenopausal or ovarian failure)

Social history

- How are you getting on at home/work? (stress/emotions)
- Do you drink/smoke/take any other substances, and how much? (substance abuse)

5

Infertility

Mr and Mrs Brown have been referred for investigation of infertility. Please take a history from each of them.

Answer follows . . .

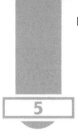

5

Infertility

Key points

Practise putting the following points into dialogue.

In answering this topic, you will need to discuss both male and female sub-fertility.

Start by introducing yourself to the couple. Ask how long they have been together and how long they have been trying for a baby. Find out if it is primary (never conceived) or secondary (have conceived before) sub-fertility for the female partner, male partner or for the couple. If they have conceived before in previous relationships find out the total number of pregnancies they have had and their outcomes, i.e. whether they ended in ectopics, miscarriages, terminations or live births. Also ask if these were natural or assisted conceptions. Enquire about problems in previous pregnancies, details of children and any history of familial hereditary disorders and genetic disorders.

A detailed menstrual history is a must when taking an infertility history from the female partner. This includes history of menarche, whether the cycles are regular/irregular and the length of cycles. You also have to ask about previous contraception history. Remember women with an IUCD are more prone to PID. Also ask about any intermenstrual bleeding and post-coital bleeding. You have to take a detailed sexual history (from both partners), such as frequency of intercourse, any pain during intercourse, any mechanical problems (e.g. erectile impotence), weight disorders and hirsutism (polycystic ovary syndrome, PCOS). Remember to ask about a previous history of any tubal or ovarian surgery, STD, PID and any medical conditions such as diabetes and thyroid disorders. Make a note of whether she has been diagnosed with endometriosis in the past. Enquire about the use of medicines that might suppress fertility, e.g. the use of diuretics may cause erectile impotence.

While taking a history for male fertility it is important to ask whether the patient has suffered in the past from a GU infection, mumps, STD, TB, torsion of the testis/testicular trauma, testicular tumours and diabetes. Undescended testes will need to be ruled out in the subsequent examination.

It is also important to make a note of the couple's social history, such as whether they smoke and how many units of alcohol they consume. Lastly, enquire about the couple's professions – some occupations involve working in very high temperatures which can suppress spermatogenesis.

End your conversation by thanking the couple and wishing them good luck.

6

Weight loss

A 16-year-old young woman has recently sustained weight loss. Please take a history and state your differential diagnosis.

Answer follows . . .

6

Weight loss

Key points
- Introduce yourself to the patient.
- Confirm the patient's idea of 'weight loss' by asking the patient:
  - When and how did you first notice this weight loss?
  - What was your weight before? How much is your weight now?
  - **Note:** a significant weight loss is defined as a loss of more than 10% of body weight over 6 months.
- Work through your differential diagnoses.
- Bear social factors in mind when taking the patient's history.
- Thank the patient.
- Be ready to quickly state your differential diagnoses.

Questions to ask the patient
Medical causes of weight loss
- Have you had a recent cough/SOB/sputum? (chest infection/TB)
- Have you any tummy pain/frequent bowel motions/vomiting? (viral illness/gastroenteritis)
- Have you noticed any blood/mucus in your motions? (inflammatory bowel disease)
- Have you noticed that the stool is difficult to flush away/clay-coloured? (malabsorption syndromes)
- Have you noticed any altered bowel habit/blood in your stool? (malignancy)

- Have you noticed yourself sweating more/disliking hot temperatures/a shaking in your arms? How are your periods? (thyroid)
- How do you feel in yourself? Are you doing well at school/work? Are you able to concentrate/sleep well/go out and enjoy yourself? Have you ever tried to harm yourself? (depression)
- Do you think you are overweight? Are you trying to lose weight? Do you exercise, how much exercise, what do you do? Are you on any special diet at the moment? Have you ever tried to lose weight by inducing vomiting or using laxatives? Are your periods regular? (anorexia nervosa/bulimia)
- Have you noticed you have been drinking more water recently and passing water more frequently? Is anybody in your family diabetic? (diabetes)
- Are you on any prescribed or over-the-counter medications/herbal remedies? (diuretics, laxatives, antidepressants)

Social considerations
- Are you particularly stressed at the moment? Do you have problems financially, at home/work/school, with exams/friends? (stress)
- Do you drink or smoke (how much)? Do you use any recreational drugs? (substance abuse)
- Who do you live with at home (e.g. partner/family/foster care)? Do you have good relations with them? (family problems)

Discussion

- Think of the basic investigations you might want to perform for each of the medical conditions mentioned above.
- Try to apply the above history-taking skills to the causes of weight **gain**.

7

Palpitations

Please imagine you are an SHO in a cardiology outpatients clinic when a young woman presents to you with a history of 'palpitations'. Take a history from the patient and discuss your management plans.

Answer follows . . .

Palpitations

Answer

In this scenario a medical term ('palpitation') has been used by the patient. However, it is important not to assume that she fully understands what this means, and so it should be clarified.

Consider your differential diagnosis before you begin, so you have a framework to work on. Remember to always rule out social causes and to get a good social picture of your patient.

Doctor–patient scenario

SHO: Good morning Miss Yates my name is Dr M., I am very pleased to meet you.

MISS Y.: Good morning doctor.

SHO: So what brings you to the clinic this morning?

MISS Y.: I've been suffering from palpitations on and off for quite some time now, my GP suggested this appointment. I hope you will be able to help me.

SHO: Well, I'll certainly try my best. I appreciate that these palpitations may be very frightening for you. Before we go any further, I would like to ask you what you mean by the word 'palpitations' exactly.

MISS Y.: Well, I suppose when they come, it's like a drum beating in my heart.

SHO: I see, alright. Does this drum beat fast or slow? Is it regular or irregular? Could you tap it out on the desk for me please.

(Miss Y. taps out the beat.)

SHO: Good, now I understand more clearly; these appear to be fast and irregular palpitations, would you agree with that? When do you get these palpitations? How long do they last? Do they stop on their own?

MISS Y.: There is no regularity, it could be after I run for the bus, it could be when I'm watching television. They last several minutes at a time and then just stop.

Rule out a familial cause

SHO: Does anybody else in your family suffer with anything similar to this?

MISS Y.: Not that I know of.

Rule out atrial fibrillation, SVT, Wolff–Parkinson–White (WPW) syndrome

SHO: Do you have any associated chest pain or shortness of breath? Have you ever lost consciousness ('blacked out') as a result of this?

MISS Y.: I do feel faint, but I haven't actually blacked out. I don't feel any pain or shortness of breath.

Rule out hyperthyroidism

SHO: Good. How are you in yourself? How's your appetite? Are your periods normal? How are your bowel habits? Have you noticed any recent tremors or sweating?

MISS Y.: I'm fine; I eat well; I'm on a diet actually so I've lost weight and get a little constipated sometimes, but I'm regular. My periods are as normal as ever.

Rule out drug side-effects

SHO: Okay, you're doing very well so far. Are you taking any prescribed/over-the-counter/herbal medication?

MISS Y.: Yes, I'm on the oral contraceptive pill.

SHO: Thank you. Do you drink or smoke? Do you take any recreational drugs?

MISS Y.: I'm a social drinker, I don't smoke, I don't take any drugs.

Rule out panic attacks

SHO: How are you at work/at home, are you under any stress?

MISS Y.: Not really, my work is fine, I'm happy at home.

SHO: One final question Miss Y., do you drink a lot of coffee?

MISS Y.: I don't like coffee, I prefer tea!

Closure

SHO: Good, excellent. Well Miss Y., I would like to arrange a few tests to make sure your heart is functioning OK and to try and get to the bottom of your problem. I would like to take a tracing of your heart called an ECG and see what it shows me. I may also go on to request a scan of your heart at a later date. Is that alright?

MISS Y.: Is this something I should be worried about doctor?

SHO: Well, I think it's important to take things one step at a time, let's have a look at the tracing of your heart first. I may decide to discuss it with my senior doctor, just to make sure nothing is overlooked. If anything is revealed on the ECG, we can discuss things from there.

MISS Y.: Yes, that seems reasonable. Thank you doctor.

SHO: My pleasure, do you have any further questions for me?

MISS Y.: Not at the moment.

Differential diagnosis

- Atrial fibrillation
- Wolff–Parkinson–White syndrome
- Panic attacks
- Hyperthyroidism
- Drug side-effects (e.g. beta-agonists)

- Recreational stimulants (e.g. coffee)
- Family history.

Discussion

Don't get caught into wasting time by explaining pathology in too much detail, the question asks for a history and a differential diagnosis enough for you to formulate an immediate management plan.

WPW syndrome seems reasonable, but don't be put off by a diagnosis of something so medical! It is reasonable and logical to undertake a basic investigation and then approach senior colleagues to discuss the case. At this stage, it is not entirely appropriate to start explaining WPW to the patient – it may not be her diagnosis!

Your patient wants you to be clear, easy to understand, easy to approach and for you to give a definitive plan of action so they know what is happening. All these points are addressed by the above simulated question-and-answer conversation. Stick to the basics, be confident and fluent in your approach.

8

Joint pain

A 50-year-old man, Mr Foote, is complaining of pain and swelling in his right great toe. A similar episode occurred 6 months ago; 3 months before that his left knee was affected. You are the SHO working in the rheumatology clinic, take a history and arrive at a diagnosis.

Answer follows . . .

8

Joint pain

Answer

Sometimes the cause of joint pain is obvious and little or no investigation is required to arrive at a diagnosis. However, there are many causes of joint pain and the cause may not always be clear.

The following table lists causes of mono (single) or poly (many) – arthritis

Table 2.1 Causes of mono- and polyarthritis

Monoarthritis	Polyarthritis
Septic arthritis (usually *Staph. aureus*/ strep./TB)	Viral causes (e.g. mumps, HIV, EBV)
Osteoarthritis	Rheumatoid arthritis (and acute rheumatic fever)
Trauma/haemarthrosis	Drug-induced
Gout	Gonorrhoea
Pseudogout	Psoriatic arthropathy
Tumour	
Reiter's syndrome	

Abbreviations: *Staph. aureus*, *Staphylococcus aureus*; strep., *Streptococcus spp.*; TB, tuberculosis; HIV, human immunodeficiency virus; EBV, Epstein–Barr virus.

The causes of joint pain can be further sub-divided into:
- **non-inflammatory**: e.g. trauma, degenerative joint diseases (osteoarthritis)
- **acute inflammatory**: e.g. acute gout, pseudogout, Reiter's syndrome, rheumatoid
- **haemorrhagic**: e.g. trauma, haemarthrosis, tumours
- **septic**: e.g. bacterial, viral, gonorrhoea
- **other**: e.g. drug-induced, enteropathic arthropathy, spondylarthritides, Henoch–Schönlein purpura (HSP), seronegative arthritis, psoriatic arthritis, juvenile causes, etc.

Bearing in mind the more common causes, you can now build a framework for your questions.

Remember: Always introduce yourself to the patient, listen attentively and thank the patient at the end of your questions.

Questions to ask the patient
Presenting complaint
- Please tell me all about the pain – onset, duration, type, site, radiation, aggravating/relieving features, associated features, previous episodes. Note that:
  - rheumatoid arthritis tends to be worse in the morning due to stiffness, whereas osteoarthritis is worse on movement. Inflammatory arthritis is typically associated with stiffness and pain that is worse at rest and may be improved with exercise. Non-inflammatory joint disease tends to be brought on with exercise and relieved by rest.
  - associated red, angry-looking joints indicate gout/pseudogout.
  - an associated 'hot', red, angry-looking joint with a raised systemic temperature indicates septic arthritis, particularly following a history of an open wound/surgery near or to the joint.

o recurrent episodes suggest an ongoing condition with acute exacerbations, e.g. osteoarthritis, gout, rheumatoid arthritis.
- Have you sustained any trauma to the joint recently? (haemarthrosis, septic arthritis)
- Have you recently travelled abroad; where did you go? (extramarital affairs, Reiter's syndrome/gonococcal arthritis – typically seen in young males)
- Have you been ill recently? (infection can trigger gout, a cause for sepsis of viral/bacterial origin)

Past medical history

There are many systemic associations with joint pain. Wait for the patient's answer. Some conditions to bear in mind include:
- hypothyroidism, hyperparathyroidism, acromegaly, haemochromatosis – pseudogout
- psoriasis – psoriatic arthritis, gout
- inflammatory bowel disease – enteropathic arthropathies
- ankylosing spondylitis (typically in young men), leukaemia (and other causes of seronegative arthritis)
- renal disease (cause of hyperuricaemia therefore precipitating gout)
- any recent history of surgery or trauma.

Drug history
- Have you started to take any new drugs recently? (thiazide diuretics, cytotoxics and salicylates are well known to precipitate gout)

Family history
- Is there any similar family history? (Note genetic links, e.g. HLA B27 in ankylosing spondylitis.)

Social history
- Do you drink or smoke? If so, how much? (alcohol is a

precipitant for gout)
- What sort of a diet do you consume? (red meats and fatty foods can trigger acute gout attacks, as can prolonged periods of starvation/dehydration)

Discussion

- You can apply the above history-taking technique to the original question:
  - ○ 'a 50-year-old man': this can generally eliminate causes such as Reiter's disease and ankylosing spondylitis. Also, rheumatoid arthritis is less common in men.
  - ○ 'is complaining of toe pain and swelling': inflammation with pain indicates an acute inflammatory process (e.g. acute gout, pseudogout, rheumatoid conditions)
  - ○ '3 months before that, his left knee was affected': therefore it is a monoarthritis (i.e. one joint at a time, eliminate rheumatoid arthritis) and an ongoing condition with recurrent exacerbations, e.g. gout/osteoarthritis.
- So from the question you are left with two most probable causes. After further prompting and eliminating 'Any trauma?' 'Is the toe red and angry looking?', the diagnosis is most likely to be acute gout.
- You can then ask about precipitants for acute gout, any causes of hyperuricaemia and other known triggers (e.g. recent surgery, diet, drugs, infection, starvation, dehydration, etc).
- Associated features on examination could include signs such as tophi (urate deposits found in avascular areas, e.g. pinna, tendons).
- Your advice for treatment would include lifestyle modifications with relation to alcohol, fatty foods and red-meat intake, as well as advice about avoiding

particular drugs and states of dehydration. If appropriate (obese patient), weight reduction can be encouraged.

- The diagnosis can be confirmed via aspiration of synovial fluid from the affected joint, microscopy should reveal fine needle-shaped, negatively birefringent crystals. (**Note** positively birefringent in pseudogout.)

- Immediate management in the acute phase includes an NSAID (e.g. ibuprofen), or colchicine for those who are unable to take NSAIDs. The aim is to reduce the pain and inflammation, which should take 1–2 days to abate.

- In the long term, treatment is aimed at reducing the serum urate level. Allopurinol is used, but not until 3 weeks after an acute attack. An alternative, if the patient develops side-effects to allopurinol, is a uricosuric drug (e.g. probenecid).

9

Headache

Mr Peterson is a 36-year-old man who presents to A&E with an unbearable headache. It started last night before he went to bed, but has become progressively worse today. He is on no medication and has no drug allergies. Please take a relevant history and outline the immediate management with your diagnosis in mind.

Answer follows . . .

9

Headache

Answer

As every doctor is aware, there are hundreds of causes for a headache. Often, the cause is unknown. In the PLAB exam (and in real-life situations), it is important to be able to rule out the most important causes of a headache quickly and effectively in the allotted 5 minutes. For this reason, it is most likely that only one of the more serious causes of a headache may be the diagnosis at the OSCE station. Remember this station is not a test of your most obscure knowledge of causes of a headache, it is a test to see if you can differentiate between a well patient and a critically ill patient and act accordingly.

For academic purposes, a classification of headaches is given in Table 2.2 and you are welcome to sit and think about these causes. However, for your exam preparation, it is important to know how to rule out the most important causes only.

Key points

Rule out causes from the patient's history
Subarachnoid haemorrhage
'Started with a bang, feels like I've been kicked in the head.'
- Does the patient have:
  - any neck stiffness?
  - any photophobia? (dislike of bright lights)

Table 2.2 Classification of headaches

Acute single (hours/days)	Acute recurrent (days/weeks)	Chronic (weeks/months)	Subacute (months/years)
Bacterial meningitis	Migraine	Chronic subdural	Tension
Subarachnoid haemorrhage	Episodic tension	Brain tumour	Analgesic abuse
Acute glaucoma	Trigeminal neuralgia	Brain abscess	Depression
Optic/retrobulbar neuritis	Coital headache	Temporal arteritis	
Cerebral ischaemia	Post-traumatic		
Hypertension	TMJ syndrome		
Acute sinusitis	Low CSF pressure		
Acute post-traumatic	Idiopathic intracranial hypertension		
Spontaneous dissection (cranial arteries)	Headache in HIV-infected patients		
Substance abuse/ withdrawal	Superior sagittal sinus thrombosis		
Metabolic disorder			
Migraine			
Carbon monoxide toxicity			

Abbreviations: TMJ, temporomandibular joint; CSF, cerebrospinal fluid; HIV, human immunodeficiency virus.
Adapted from Silberstein, S.D. (1992). Evaluation of the emergency treatment of headache. *Headache* 32(8), 396–407.

- any vomiting?
- any focal neurology? (weakness/numbness in any arm/leg?)

Bacterial meningitis

- Does the patient have:
  - any rash over their body? If so, do the spots blanch on pressure?
  - any neck stiffness?
  - any photophobia?
  - a sore throat/fever/ear discharge?
  - any history of travel abroad recently? Where? (possible contact/other infectious disease)

Space-occupying lesion

'The headaches are worse first thing in the morning, doctor.' 'The pain gets worse with coughing/sneezing and bending over.'

- Does the patient have:
  - any history of weight loss?
  - any history of cancer elsewhere? (rule out a primary with brain metastases)
  - any focal deficit? (weakness or numbness in a certain limb/altered speech)
  - any vomiting/visual disturbances?

Subdural haematoma (Note: this is more common in elderly people and alcoholics)

- Does the patient have:
  - any history of recent trauma?
  - 'lucid intervals' or a fluctuating level of consciousness?
  - family members who are concerned that s/he has become increasingly confused?
  - signs of an increased intracranial pressure.

Temporal arteritis/giant-cell arteritis

- This is more common in those over 55 years of age.

- Patients typically mention scalp tenderness: 'It hurts when I comb my hair, doctor'.
- Needs to be diagnosed quickly to prevent progression to sudden blindness.
- An ESR (>40 mm/h) is highly suggestive of this condition. Treatment is with high-dose steroids (e.g. 60 mg prednisolone).

Acute angle closure glaucoma (usually elderly people)

- If the patient is a younger person, rule out a family history of glaucoma.
- Does the patient have pain around one particular eye, decreased vision, vomiting?
- The patient may have a red eye. **Big clue** – pupils **not** reacting.
- Does the patient have a tender eyeball?

Previous medical history

- Does the patient have:
  - diabetes? (hypoglycaemic attack)
  - does the patient wear glasses? (need for an eye test)
  - hypertension? (but **don't** simply attribute the headache to this)
  - a history of a recent cough/cold? (sinusitis)
  - any past history of cancer? (possibility of brain metastases)

Drug history

- Has the patient:
  - recently started taking any new prescribed/over-the-counter/herbal medications? (possible side-effect)
  - recently stopped taking long-term medications? (withdrawal effect)
  - been taking the oral contraceptive pill? (small risk of superior sagittal sinus thrombosis)

Social history
- Does the patient:
  - have any stresses/worries? (tension headache, typically like a 'band' around the head)
  - demonstrate any substance abuse?
  - live alone, is he elderly, does he have a leaking heating system or new installation? (carbon monoxide poisoning)

Discussion

There is more than enough information to rule out the most sinister causes of a headache.

Try to formulate management plans and keep them ready for discussion.

10

Alcohol

Mr Drinkwater has been admitted to undergo surgery for an inguinal hernia. Pre-operative investigations reveal an increased mean corpuscular volume. You suspect he has a high alcohol intake. Take a history from him regarding his alcohol habits.

Answer follows . . .

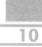

10

Alcohol

Answer

Alcohol abuse is a worldwide problem, and is especially recognised in the Western world. It is important to know how to deal with this as you will come across such patients in your work fairly frequently. In this case scenario the patient has presented to you with an unrelated problem, so broaching the subject may be difficult.

It is important to distinguish heavy drinking (an alcohol intake in excess of the recommended levels) from alcoholism (an actual dependency on alcohol with withdrawal symptoms on abstinence). The following mnemonics are useful aids when communicating with the patient:

'CONTROL'
- Can you always **CO**ntrol your drinking?
- Has alcohol ever led you to **N**eglect your family/job?
- What **T**ime do you start drinking?
- Have friends ever asked you to **R**educe your alcohol intake?
- Do you ever drink in the mornings to **O**vercome a hangover?
- Go through an average day's alcohol intake **L**eaving nothing out.

'CAGE' (three or more positive answers is significant)
- Have you ever tried to **C**ut down your drinking?
- Do you ever get **A**ngry when people talk to you about

your drinking?
- Do you ever feel **G**uilty about your drinking?
- Do you ever have a drink first thing in the morning? (an **E**ye-opener)

Questions to ask the patient

Alcohol intake

- How much would you have to drink during an average week? (One unit is the equivalent of a shot of spirit, a small glass of wine or half a pint of beer. Women are allowed 7–14 units a week; men are allowed 14–21 units a week.)
- What exactly do you like to drink (spirits/beer/lager, etc)?
- Do you drink with friends or alone?
- Does your drinking follow a pattern or is it binge drinking?

Social background

Heavy drinking, with its attendant repercussions, is generally triggered by one or more factors. Ask about:
- job performance (recent change in job or redundancy)
- family life (marital status, child abuse, financial difficulties)
- any convictions for drink driving
- whether **either** parent is/was a heavy drinker, since alcoholism is often familial.

Patient awareness

This is a most important and sensitive area. Does the patient know he has a problem? Has he tried to help himself previously?
- Features of alcohol dependence include withdrawal symptoms (delirium tremens), usually first thing in the morning. Does the patient have 'an eye opener' to help start the day?

- Has he noticed that he needs more and more alcohol to reach the same level of satisfaction?
- Does he sometimes have hallucinations? Classically, visual hallucinations take the form of insects or brightly coloured animals – 'pink elephants'.
- Is he aware that he consumes too much alcohol and has he tried to cut down in the past? If so, was it through detoxification programmes, joining Alcoholics Anonymous (AA) or visiting his GP to ask for advice?

Discussion

Health problems associated with alcoholism
- Liver cirrhosis
- Portal hypertension
- Haematemesis
- Peptic ulcer disease
- Pancreatitis
- Ischaemic heart disease
- Stroke
- Epilepsy
- Malnutrition
- Ataxia, peripheral neuropathy
- Psychiatric problems (anxiety, hallucinations, depression, Korsakoff's psychosis, Wernicke's encephalopathy)
- Head injury
- Impotence.

What is Pabrinex?
Pabrinex is the trade name for a high-potency, parenteral preparation of vitamins B and C, including vitamin B_1 (i.e. thiamine).
- Given to patients in an alcohol coma or those with an alcohol-induced psychosis, it can help to reverse the condition by correcting the severe vitamin depletion.

What is chlordiazepoxide?

Librium is one trade name. This is an oral regime, given to help patients with symptoms of moderate to severe alcohol withdrawal. It can help ameliorate tremors and hallucinations, and also has a sedative action. An alternative is diazepam (Valium).

- These days, clomethiazole (chlormethiazole) is rarely used because of the risk of respiratory depression.

11

Fever

Mr Richter is a 27-year-old man who has recently been travelling in the Far East (on business). He presents to you feeling generally unwell and has been pyrexial for the past 5 days. Please take a history and establish a list of possible differential diagnoses.

Answer follows . . .

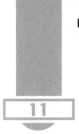

11

Fever

Answer

This is usually a history-taking station.

Remember: always introduce yourself to the patient and thank them at the end of the exam.

Questions to ask the patient

- Determine the patient's symptoms of 'fever' (i.e. chills and rigors, sweating, feeling lethargic), ask the patient:
  - When did it start?
  - Is it getting worse or better?
  - Have you taken your temperature?
  - Also ask about symptoms of a viral illness, which can include myalgia, feeling of lethargy, runny nose.
- Attempt to determine the focus of infection:
  - **Chest**:
  - Have you had a cough/sputum, what colour is the sputum, have you noticed any blood?
  - Have you had any recent contact with TB?
  - Have you any chest pain? (rule out pleuritic causes)
  - Do you smoke? If so, how many?
  - **Gastrointestinal**:
  - Are your bowels working normally?
  - Have you had any diarrhoea? Have you passed blood/mucus from your rectum?
  - Have you recently had a meal in a restaurant or from a take-away?

- ○ Is anybody else in the family affected? (rule out gastroenteritis/inflammatory bowel disease)
- ○ Have you travelled abroad recently? (consider infectious diseases, e.g. malaria)
- ○ Have you noticed any jaundice? (rule out hepatitis)
- ○ Have you lost any weight? (chronic problems)
- ○ Do you drink alcohol? If so, how much?
- ○ **Cardiac**:
- ○ Do you have any chest pain?
- ○ Have you any history of rheumatic heart disease?
- ○ **Neurological**:
- ○ Do you have a headache/photophobia or neck stiffness? (rule out meningitis)
- ○ **Genitourinary**:
- ○ Have you dysuria, any lower abdominal/loin pain? (rule out UTI/pyelonephritis)
- ○ Have you noticed any discharge from 'down below' (perineum)? (STD)
- ○ **Skin**:
- ○ Have you noticed any redness or a painful rash?
- If the above history is negative, think of other possibilities (the initial question should guide you), ask:
  - ○ Have you had any recent vaccinations, e.g. 'flu jab'? (which **cannot** cause flu, but may be followed by a brief pyrexia)
  - ○ Have you an abscess or wound? (i.e. a localised focus)
  - ○ What are your social circumstances? (ask with sensitivity; e.g. is the patient an iv drug abuser?)

Discussion

Question: What basic investigations might you proceed to conduct if no definite diagnosis was available?

Answer: Full blood count, C-reactive protein (CRP), blood cultures, mid-stream urinalysis (MSU), chest X-ray, sputum or stool culture (if appropriate).

Question: If the patient was an inpatient presenting with pyrexia, what might you do?

Answer: A thorough examination would be required. I would first re-check the patient's temperature (core temperature with a reliable thermometer). I would examine any peripheral access sites, e.g. cannulas (possibly causing thrombophlebitis) and any catheters (which may harbour infection). I would listen to the heart for any new murmurs (bacterial endocarditis), and to the chest for any crepitations (chest infection). It would then be important to consider the same basic investigations as above, I would document all findings in the patient's notes.

Note: Take time out to consider the pyrexial patient in special circumstances:
• the post-operative patient
• the neutropenic patient
• a patient with HIV
• an iv drug abuser.

It is important to run through some variants in your own mind, so if a question is thrown at you out of the blue, you **will** be prepared for it!

12

Haematuria

Please imagine you are the SHO working in a urology clinic. A 43-year-old man, Mr Khan, presents to you with a history of passing blood in his water. Please take a history and present your differential diagnoses at the end.

Answer follows . . .

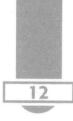

12

Haematuria

Answer

This station focuses entirely on your history-taking skills. Use the full 4 min and 30 s to obtain a good history, so by the time the 30-s bell pings you can rattle off your differential diagnoses.

Remember:

- to keep differential diagnoses in mind so you can focus your questions
- to introduce yourself to the patient and to thank him at the end.

Doctor–patient scenario

Introduction

SHO: Good afternoon Mr Khan, how can I help you today?

MR K.: Doctor, I'm really quite worried, there seems to be blood in my water, it's been going on for a few months now.

SHO: Yes, I can understand this must be quite disconcerting for you.

Determine the likely site of bleeding

SHO: Mr K., is the bleeding at the start of the stream (urethra), throughout the stream (bladder/ureter/kidney) or at the end of the stream (prostate/base of bladder)?

MR K.: I'm not really sure, I think it's throughout, mixed with the urine.

Rule out trauma

SHO: Right, Mr K., do you remember sustaining any injury to your private parts, or your tummy?

MR K.: No.

Rule out infection

SHO: Good. Do you notice any burning sensation when you pass water, or pain in your lower tummy? Have you noticed a fever or any discharge from your penis?

MR K.: I think I get a fever sometimes. No burning or pain. No discharge.

Rule out prostatic problems

SHO: I see, have you noticed any change in the frequency or amount of water you pass, how is the stream itself?

MR K.: The stream is fine. Nothing has changed, except the blood.

SHO: Have you ever been incontinent of urine?

MR K.: No.

Rule out carcinoma

SHO: Where do you work Mr K.?

MR K.: On a market stall.

SHO: Have you noticed any weight loss recently?

MR K.: Yes, I think I have lost some weight.

Rule out renal calculi

SHO: Have you any history of stones or passing a stone?

MR K.: No.

SHO: Do you ever have an urge to pass water without a result?

MR K.: No.

Rule out bleeding diathesis

SHO: Do you bleed from any other sites, e.g. your nose, ears, etc?

MR K.: Not really, no.

Rule out drug side-effects

SHO: Are you on any medications?

MR K.: I take paracetamol for headaches sometimes.

Past medical history

SHO: Are you fit and well in yourself?

MR K.: I've been having a bit of a cough recently, just won't go away. I've been feeling tired, you know, not my usual self.

Rule out infectious disease

SHO: Have you travelled abroad recently?

MR K.: I went to visit my mother in Pakistan, but that was a few months ago.

SHO: Do you drink or smoke, sir?

MR K.: Neither.

Differential diagnoses

- Trauma
- Malignancy
- UTI
- Renal calculi
- Bleeding diathesis
- Side-effects of medications
- Infectious diseases, including TB.

Discussion

If there is time the examiner may probe further, so know why you are asking your questions!

Question: Why did you ask about medications?

Answer: Rifampicin can colour the body fluids a reddish colour. Sulfasalazine (sulphasalazine) can colour urine orange. L-Dopa can colour urine red. Warfarin may result in bleeding problems. (**Note**: Lots of beetroot can also colour the urine red!)

Question: Why did you ask Mr K. where he worked?

Answer: There is a known link between workers in rubber factories or aniline dyeworks and the development of bladder carcinoma.

Question: Why did you ask about travel abroad?

Answer: To rule out infectious diseases such as schistosomiasis and tuberculosis, I feel the latter may be the case in this patient.

13

Diarrhoea

Please imagine you are an SHO in the outpatients surgical clinic. A 47-year-old man, Mr Loosemoore, has presented to you complaining of diarrhoea. Please elicit a history and discuss the differential diagnosis.

Answer follows . . .

13

Diarrhoea

Answer

- Consider your differential diagnosis beforehand, to use as a framework for your discussion:
  - traveller's diarrhoea/infective cause
  - thyrotoxicosis
  - autonomic neuropathy (diabetes mellitus)
  - drug-induced (antibiotics, also rule out *Clostridium difficile* infection)
  - malignancy
  - inflammatory bowel disease
  - irritable bowel syndrome.

- Remember to introduce yourself to the patient, maintain a relaxed atmosphere in this potentially embarrassing situation for the patient and to thank him at the end of the station.
- Establish what the patient means by the term 'diarrhoea' – it may mean increased stool frequency, liquidity, or both. How many times does he normally open his bowels in a day? How long has this change in bowel habit been noticed?
- Ask the patient to describe the diarrhoea itself: colour, consistency, odour, any blood/mucus, episodes per day?
- Rule out your differential diagnoses.

Questions to ask the patient

Rule out traveller's diarrhoea/infective causes

- Have you eaten out in a restaurant recently or had a

take-away? How are other family members?
- Any history of travel abroad? Where did you go? When did you get back? Where did you stay? What food did you eat?
- Have you noticed a fever?

Rule out thyrotoxicosis
- Have you noticed any changes in yourself, are you more nervous than usual?
- Have you noticed a particular dislike for hot weather?
- Have you noticed any shakiness/sweating?
- Have you lost any weight?
- (if female, how are your periods?)

Rule out autonomic neuropathy
- Are you a diabetic? Have you had your blood sugar checked recently?
- If diagnosed – what medications are you taking? Have you noticed a decreased sensation in your legs? Do you feel dizzy after standing up too quickly? Do you find it difficult to get your balance on occasions?

Rule out drug-induced diarrhoea
- Are you on any medication? Have you recently started or finished a course of antibiotics?

Rule out malignancy
- Have you noticed any weight loss? How much over how long?
- Have you noticed any blood in your stool? Have you noticed your bowel habit to alternate between constipation and diarrhoea? Do you sometimes find that you have the urge to pass stool but don't get a result?
- Do you have a family history of any type of cancer?
- Are you fit and well in yourself?

Rule out inflammatory bowel disease
- Have you had similar episodes of diarrhoea in the past on and off?
- Do you have any other medical problems?
- Do you have any back pain, joint problems or eye problems?
- Does anybody in your family have any similar problems?
- Have you noticed any blood or mucous in the stool?
- Have you lost weight recently?
- Do you sometimes feel tummy pain when you want to pass a stool?

Rule out irritable bowel disease
- Do you have a lot of stress in your life at the moment?
- Have you noticed this diarrhoea gets worse at certain times in your life? If so, when?
- Do you also feel bloated when you get this problem?
- Would you say you are an anxious person?
- What have you tried for this problem?
- Do you sometimes have pellet-like stools?

Discussion

Obviously it may not be necessary to ask so many questions for each differential diagnosis. If the patient answers 'No' to a certain question there is often no need to proceed any further and you proceed to the next differential.

A note on drugs

Various drugs may result in diarrhoea – antibiotics are well known. Keep a few more in mind, e.g. propanolol, cimetidine, metformin, statins.

It is important to be aware of the possibility of *Clostridium difficile* infection, which is iatrogenic due to long-term antibiotic therapy.

Inflammatory bowel disease

Generally, this is more likely if the candidate is young and male, or with a positive family history.

14

Child abuse

Imagine you are the SHO on a paediatric ward. While examining a 4-month-old baby for a respiratory infection you notice bruises on its ear. Please take a history from the mother of how the baby sustained these bruises and say how you would proceed in this case.

Answer follows . . .

14

Child abuse

Answer

At any one time 2% of the UK child population is a victim of child abuse. A third of these will be sexual abuse cases.

When talking to a parent/carer/child you should always bear in mind the possibility of child abuse. What you see is likely to be as important as what you are told in the history.

Things to look out for include the child's mental alertness to their surroundings – at the extreme described as: frozen awareness; hypervigilance; increased appetite and disturbed feeding behaviours; and decreased interpersonal interactions. Remember that children with learning difficulties may be at a greater risk of abuse. Even if a child is clinging strongly to its mother, this does not rule out the possibility of abuse.

Parental factors associated with abuse include a known history of abuse to the parent, chronic medical problems, severe depression/neurotic disorders and substance abuse. Poor social support or financial difficulties also present a risk.

Points to consider in the history and examination

- An inconsistent history between parents, or one that changes each time.
- A delay between the injury and when help is sought.
- An inappropriate explanation as to how the injury occurred – for example:

YOU: OK Mrs B., I've had a listen to his chest and I think it's just a viral infection which will probably clear up in a week. He seems to be over the worst of it now, which is good news. However, while examining him I noticed some marks on his ear – they look like old bruises. Can you tell me how he got these bruises?

MOTHER: Oh, they happened when he rolled off the sofa.

YOU: How long ago was that?

MOTHER: It must be about a week ago now. He must have landed on his ear I suppose.

YOU: Did you get them looked at?

MOTHER: They didn't seem to bother him much.

YOU: What were you doing at the time?

MOTHER: I was in the kitchen. His older brother was in the room with him, but he's only four. I suppose he may have done it.

YOU: Caused the bruises you mean? What about the fall off the sofa – didn't you think that may have caused the bruises?

MOTHER: I'm not sure. I think so. His brother might have pulled him off the sofa too. I'm not sure how it may have happened.

YOU: Did he cry immediately after falling?

MOTHER: Not much more than usual.

YOU: Is he usually quite accident prone? Does he come to hospital often?

MOTHER: He doesn't come to hospital often. Though I suppose he often gets bumps and bruises, but it's normal for a child his age isn't it?

YOU: Well, it can be, but he's still a little young for crawling and exploring. Does he have any blood disorders that you know of – does he bruise easily? And how are things between him and his brother?

MOTHER: Nothing that I know of for the blood. His brother loves to play with him, pesters him all day!

YOU: Okay. Where's his father at the moment?

MOTHER: He's at work.

YOU: And his brother?

MOTHER: At home.

YOU: By himself?

MOTHER: Yes. Why?

YOU: Is he usually alright by himself? Is there any reason you didn't bring him?

MOTHER: Well this one's enough of a handful, so I told him to wait for me to get back.

(*There are several inconsistencies in this story. First, a 4-month-old baby cannot roll over, and cannot walk or crawl so bruises are uncommon. Second, there has been a delay between the injury occurring and getting help. Falling off a sofa, and presumably landing on a carpet, is unlikely to cause bruising to the ear – which is itself an uncommon site for accidental injury. The mother's story changes, from saying the baby fell to blaming the older brother, which is also suspicious. It also seems to be a little irresponsible to leave a 4-year-old child alone. Such a case should set off alarm bells in your head, although it would also be a good idea to speak to the father, if possible. However, it is important not to accuse anyone of anything at this time. You do not want to offend the parents as the protection and treatment of a child becomes difficult if there is parental resistance.*)

YOU: Thanks for all the answers you've given. I'm sorry, but I'm not happy with the explanation you have given me about your son's bruises. I would like to call some other members of my team to take another look at him if that's OK with you . . .

Features to look for in any history and examination

- While bruising is common in an active child, they tend to occur on bony prominences such as the elbows, shins and forehead. Be suspicious of any well-protected areas such as the ear, the back or abdomen and inner thighs.

The latter is more suggestive of sexual abuse.
- Adult or animal bite marks need to be explained.
- A baby presenting with impaired consciousness may have been shaken, leading to a subdural haematoma. In such cases, remember to look in its eyes for retinal haemorrhages.
- Cigarette burns are usually symmetrical and circular. They are often 'explained' as splash burns, though these tend to be on exposed parts and are less perfectly circular. The shapes of burns can suggest the instrument used, for example an iron. Scald marks on both feet suggest the child was forcibly held in hot water. There may also be a circular patch over the bottom as the child draws up its feet. The explanation given may be that the child walked into the bath unattended – in which case the burn would probably be over one leg only.
- Fractures are not uncommon in children. However, a child who cannot walk is unlikely to fracture a leg. Suspicious presentations include pain in a limb (with the infant or child being reluctant to move that limb) and multiple fractures at different stages of healing. Spiral fractures are suggestive of a limb being twisted. Rib fractures from crushing tend to be posterior. Epiphyseal fractures occur from pulling on a limb.

Other types of abuse
Remember, physical abuse is only one category of abuse. Other types of abuse may take the form of neglect, emotional abuse and sexual abuse.

Neglect
There are five components to neglectful parenting:
- refusing a child's medical needs
- gross safety neglect due to a lack of safety or supervision
- emotional deprivation
- educational neglect – depends on local laws, but is

generally defined as persistent non-attendance at school without adequate explanation
- physical neglect – inadequate food, clothing or shelter resulting in harm to normal development.

Emotional abuse

Examples of emotional abuse include neglect, rejection, gross overprotection, verbal abuse and scapegoating. It may be hard to identify. Often the only presentation may be that of non-organic failure to thrive, which can be one of the earliest indications of serious parent/child interaction dysfunction. Usually the child's growth is inhibited in the home environment while it shows a normal (or above normal) growth velocity when placed out of the home, e.g. in hospital or in alternative care. It is caused by caloric deprivation accompanied by emotional deprivation.

Sexual abuse

Remember it is not only relatives who can sexually abuse a child. Any act of a sexual nature – such as sexual contact with the child's genitals or anal area, or, for example, seminal ejaculation which comes into contact with the child's skin – is an act of abuse. Sexual contact may be made by hand, mouth and genital organs. Sexual abuse also includes involving children in the production and/or consumption of pornographic material.

Investigations

When you become suspicious, it is your duty to inform the duty social worker or contact the parents' social worker if they are known to the authorities. The child may already be on the 'At-risk Register', or need placing on it. A further history may be taken by the social worker. You should also contact your registrar or consultant.

Investigations that may need your attention include:

- a clotting screen (full blood count, including platelets) to rule out blood dyscrasias (this is mandatory in any case of suspected physical abuse)
- blood biochemistry (including bone)
- a full skeletal survey – radiology of the whole skeleton to look for old or undiagnosed fractures may be needed.

Also consider medical photography of any affected area.

Documentation

Good note-taking – date and time, clarity of report, people present, signature and grade – are particularly important as cases can end in court. Black ink should be used in case the notes have to be photocopied. Include the dates and times of all events and record any inconsistencies in your history notes.

A clear, dispassionate description of any physical findings, preferably accompanied by a witnessed photograph, is needed.

Junior staff should note examination findings as they see them, but not speculate as to how they occurred.

Trauma and orthopaedics

1

Assessment of the Glasgow Coma Scale (GCS)

An 18-year-old young man is brought to A&E where you are working as an SHO. His mother says that he has had 'flu for a day and had complained of a headache. He is no longer responding to her. On examination, he has a temperature of 38.0 °C, neck stiffness and a sparse non-blanching rash over his chest. He responds to verbal stimulation by opening his eyes and speaking in a confused manner.

1. What is the most likely diagnosis?
2. What is his Glasgow Coma Scale score?
3. What treatment would you institute immediately?

Answer follows . . .

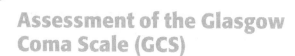

Assessment of the Glasgow Coma Scale (GCS)

Answer

1. The most likely diagnosis is meningococcal meningitis. This is a true emergency and treatment must instituted as soon as possible. Do not delay treatment while waiting for the results of blood tests or obtaining cerebrospinal fluid samples. Mortality and morbidity are high even with prompt treatment.

2. The Glasgow Coma Scale is used to assess the depth of coma (Table 3.1). In this case: Eye response, 3; Verbal response, 4; Motor response, 6; Total, 13.

3. The immediate treatment is intravenous 1.2 g benzylpenicillin or 2 g cefotaxime. Other important management strategies include intravenous fluids, and possibly steroids. Contact tracing of close contacts will be required and these people should receive antibiotic prophylaxis (usually rifampicin).

Table 3.1 Glasgow Coma Scale

System	Response	Score
Eye	Opens spontaneously	4
	Opens to command	3
	Opens to pain	2
	Does not open	1
Verbal	Talking and orientated	5
	Confused speech	4
	Inappropriate words	3
	Incomprehensible sounds	2
	No response	1
Motor	Obeys commands	6
	Localises pain	5
	Flexion/withdrawal	4
	Abnormal flexion	3
	Extension	2
	No response	1
	Total score	3–15

2

Primary survey

You are called to the ward urgently to see a 45-year-old patient who has become very ill. When you arrive you see that this man is responsive to painful stimuli, but will not respond to voice. He is clearly very ill.

Describe what initial actions you would take to assess this man.

Answer follows . . .

2

Primary survey

Answer

The initial approach for any critically ill patient is the same regardless of the cause of their illness.

Call for help

A very ill patient needs to be treated by more than one doctor. Consider calling the cardiac arrest team if cardiac or respiratory arrest looks imminent.

Airway

- Is the airway clear?
- Listen for noisy breathing, which might indicate partial airway obstruction.
- Give the patient oxygen by mask. Look at the oxygen mask to see if the mask is misting, indicating at least some expiratory effort.
- If the airway appears obstructed try to open it, use a jaw thrust or a chin lift.
- Airway adjuncts, such as a nasopharyngeal tube or a Guedel airway, may be helpful.

Breathing

- Is the patient breathing?
- Is he cyanosed?
- What is his respiratory rate?
- Are both sides of his chest moving, and can you hear breath sounds on both sides of his chest?

- If he is not breathing, or his respiratory effort is very low, he may require assisted ventilation by mouth to mouth or by a bag valve mask device.
- Pulse oximetry to record his oxygen saturation levels is helpful.

Circulation

- Does he have a pulse? What is the rate?
- What is his blood pressure?
- Consider whether his skin is well perfused by using the capillary refill time. (Press on a central point for 5 s and see how long it takes for colour to come back to the white area, longer than 2 s is abnormal.)
- Examine his neck veins to look for venous distension, indicating fluid overload or pericardial constriction.
- Empty neck veins indicate volume depletion. Attach a cardiac monitor. Look for a source of bleeding in the abdomen or rectum. Insert a venous cannula and measure his blood glucose level at the bedside.

Disability

- Only move onto this step when you have control of the airway, breathing and circulation.
- Assess the level of response using the AVPU scale (**A**lert, **V**erbal, **P**ainful, **U**nresponsive) and the Glasgow Coma Scale.
- Perform a full neurological examination, paying particular attention to the pupils, asymmetry of reflexes and muscle tone.

Exposure

- Fully examine the other body systems to look for underlying causes of this patient's illness.

3

Secondary survey

A 38-year-old man fell off his motorbike and has sustained multiple injuries. He is given high-flow oxygen and can protect his own airway. His neck is immobilised and bilateral tube thoracostomies have been inserted for pneumothoraces. His blood pressure and pulse rate are within normal limits. He is unable to communicate with you verbally because of a head injury, but moans to pain.

Describe your systems for picking up other injuries and for further evaluation.

Answer follows . . .

3

Secondary survey

Answer

- He should undergo a full secondary survey. His GCS should be recorded and a mini-neurological examination performed. This records his pupil size, the presence or absence of haemotypanums, peripheral tone and reflexes bilaterally. The semi-rigid collar should only be removed if someone else can maintain immobilisation for you.
- The scalp should be inspected for lacerations: these should be digitally explored (while wearing sterile gloves).
- The mouth should be examined and any missing teeth accounted for. Consider whether a tooth may have been aspirated.
- The neck should be inspected for lacerations and haematomas.
- The patient should be fully exposed and any areas of bruising or lacerations recorded.
- The chest and abdomen should be re-examined and the pelvis 'sprung' once.
- The external genitalia should be inspected for scrotal haematomas and blood at the meatus, indicating damage to the urogenital tract. In women, a vaginal examination is necessary.
- The upper limbs should be inspected, palpated and moved. Any areas of tenderness should be X-rayed.
- The lower limbs should also inspected, palpated and moved. Any areas of tenderness should be X-rayed.

- The patient should be log-rolled and his back inspected for haematomas. The spinal column should be palpated for tenderness or crepitus.
- A rectal examination should be performed: consider the anal tone, presence of palpable fractures.
- An attempt should be made to find out whether the patient has any allergies, takes regular medication (either prescribed or bought over the counter), has any current or previous medical problems and when he last ate.

4

Examination of the hip

A 14-year-old boy is brought to you complaining of a painful hip. This happened 2 days ago while he was getting out of a chair, and he has since walked with a limp. He has been seen by his GP a couple of times before because his mother was concerned that he was too fat, but there is no other medical history.

1. Describe how you would examine this boy's hip.
2. What is the most likely diagnosis?
3. What would you say to the boy and his mother?

Answer follows . . .

4

Examination of the hip

Answer

1. Examination:
   - **Look**: at the general state of the boy. Is he obese and/or hypogonadal? Inspect his legs to see if there is any shortening or rotation.
   - **Feel**: if there are hot or inflamed areas in the region of the greater trochanter.
   - **Move**: to assess: flexion (hold the iliac crest to prevent rotation of the pelvis); abduction (place your hand between the iliac spines to prevent pelvic tilt); abduction in flexion; adduction; and internal and external rotation. Use the Trendelenberg test to assess the stability of the pelvis and Thomas' test to assess for a fixed flexion deformity. Consider the possibility of neurological or vascular problems. Finally, if the patient is not in significant pain, ask them to walk away from and back to you.

2. A slipped upper femoral epiphysis is the most likely diagnosis.

3. I would explain that the growth plate has slipped off the top of his hip. If this is untreated it can result in deformity. An operation to place pins to hold the femoral head is recommended for minor slips. Larger slips may require more complex surgery. Once one upper femoral epiphysis has slipped the other hip is likely to slip, and surveillance is recommended. However, some surgeons may recommend prophylactic pinning of the other hip.

5

Examination of the knee

A 72-year-old woman comes to see you (her GP) complaining of a painful knee. Over the last 2 years she has suffered increasing pain and stiffness in her left knee. The pain has been so bad that she has been unable to sleep at night. She finds the pain much worse in the morning, and has noticed that the knee swells at the end of the day. She finds walking difficult. In her early twenties she broke her leg in a car accident and was in plaster for several months. She has no other joint pains. She has a past medical history of hypertension and peptic ulcer disease.

1. *Describe how you would examine this patient's knee.*
2. *What is the most likely diagnosis?*

Answer follows . . .

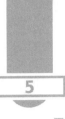

5

Examination of the knee

Answer

1. Compare both sides.
   - **Look**: The knees should be inspected for swelling, redness, scars and deformity. The quadriceps muscles should inspected for wasting.
   - **Feel**: Ask the patient to let you know if there is any pain in her knee. The knee should be palpated for warmth and the presence of an effusion. One way of demonstrating a knee effusion is to place a hand over the suprapatellar pouch and tap the patellar down onto the femur. A 'knock' will be felt with only 30 ml of fluid.
   - **Move**: Active movements should be assessed first. Flexion and extension should be compared. Ligamentous laxity should be assessed. The medial collateral ligament should be stressed by placing one hand on the outside of the thigh and lifting the ankle just off the couch so the leg is just flexed. The leg should be moved into valgus. Reversing the strains tests the lateral collateral. The cruciate ligaments are assessed by placing both the patient's feet flat on the couch with her knees flexed to 90°, then sitting on her feet (asking the patient's permission first). Placing both hands around the top of the leg with the fingers interlocking and thumbs on the femoral condyles, pull and push the leg. Excessive anterior glide indicates anterior cruciate weakness, and excessive posterior

glide indicates posterior cruciate weakness.

○   The integrity of the meniscal cartilages should be assessed by McMurray's test. The patient should be warned in advance that this test may be painful! The test is performed by flexing the knee and laterally rotating the tibia on the femur. This is repeated in various degrees of extension. The procedure is then repeated with the tibia medially rotated. The test is positive if there is a click and a pain in the knee as the leg is straightened.

2. Pain and stiffness that is much worse in the morning suggests an arthritic process. Swelling in the evening is also consistent with arthritis. Previously fractured joints are likely to develop secondary osteoarthritis. This is the most likely diagnosis in this case. (Remember that pain in the knee may be referred from the hip.)

6

Examination of the shoulder

A 35-year-old man comes to see you wanting advice about his shoulder. Some 6 months ago he fell off his bicycle and fractured his clavicle. He wore a sling for 2 months. His pain has now resolved. Now he is keen to return to climbing, but wonders whether his shoulder movements are adequate.

Describe how you would examine this man's shoulder.

Answer follows . . .

6

Examination of the shoulder

Answer

- **Look** at the shoulder joint. Is there any wasting around the muscles of the shoulder?
- **Feel** the shoulder, are there any warm or tender areas?
- **Move** the shoulder. It is best to start with active movements first and to compare with the other shoulder. Specifically assess whether there is any restriction of: flexion (forward movement); extension (ask the patient to push his elbows backwards); abduction; adduction; and medial and lateral rotation. To assess medial rotation of the shoulder ask the patient to put both hands on his back and push his elbows forward. Lateral rotation is assessed by asking the patient to put his elbows by his sides and letting his hands go out to the sides.
- If active movements are full then there is no need to perform passive movements of the shoulder.

7

Examination of the spine

A 55-year-old man presents with a sudden onset of low back pain. Outline how you would evaluate this man.

Low back pain is extremely common and it is very likely that you will see patients with this problem.

Answer follows . . .

7

Examination of the spine

Answer

History

- The onset of the pain should be described.
- He should be asked what he was doing when the pain started, e.g. lifting heavy boxes. Trauma might suggest the need for X-rays.
- The location, nature and radiation of the pain should be recorded, specifically whether the pain radiates down one or both legs.
- Exacerbating and relieving factors should be identified, e.g. sneezing or straining.
- The presence of pain in other joints is suggestive of arthritis.
- The patient's mobility should be assessed and a social and occupational history taken.
- Medications, particularly analgesics and their effect, should be recorded. He should be asked whether he is allergic to any medications.

Examination

- The **back** should be visually inspected for deformity or areas of inflammation. The vertebrae should be palpated to identify bony tenderness. The movements of the back should be assessed with the patient standing. Forward flexion should be assessed by Schrober's test. This assesses how much movement there is at the lumbar vertebrae. A tape measure is placed between two vertebrae and the patient asked to lean forward as if touching their toes. The distance between the two vertebrae is re-measured. An unchanged distance implies reduced forward flexion at the lumbar vertebrae. Lateral rotation and lateral flexion requires that the hips are fixed in position. The patient is then asked to lie down. Straight-leg raising should be performed to identify whether there is any nerve root irritation.

- The **abdomen** should be examined in the standard manner, in particular to decide whether there is an aortic aneurysm.
- The **legs** should be examined neurologically and a rectal examination may be necessary if a spinal cord or cauda equina lesion is suspected.

Investigations

These will depend on the history and examination findings.

- X-rays are necessary if there has been a history of trauma, but are probably unnecessary in a patient with no history of trauma unless there are neurological symptoms and signs. A radio-isotope bone scan is indicated if malignancy is suspected.
- Urinalysis is easy and cheap and should be done. The presence of haematuria should prompt further investigation in the urinary tract.
- Inflammatory markers, such as the erythrocyte sedimentation rate (ESR), C-reactive protein (CRP) level and white cell count, should be requested if an inflammatory or malignant cause is suspected. HLA status may be useful if ankylosing spondylitis is considered.
- In older people, an osteoporotic vertebral crush fracture can occur with minimal or no trauma.

Remember that carcinoma of the prostate and multiple myeloma often present with no pain.

8

Colles' fracture (1)

An 86-year old woman is brought to you, the SHO in Emergency Medicine, having had a fall. She complains of a sore wrist. An X-ray demonstrates an undisplaced fracture of the distal radius.

Describe how you would evaluate this woman.

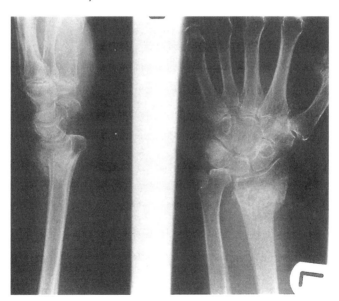

Figure 3.1

8

Colles' fracture (1)

Answer

History

- The circumstances of the fall should be described, which may require witnesses. In particular, it must be determined whether this was a simple trip (mechanical fall) or whether there is an underlying medical problem. Specific enquiries should be made about loss of consciousness, amnesia, palpitations, chest pain, confusion and fitting. You should ask if she's recently had new glasses (e.g. bifocals) or an eye test (she may need a new prescription, has developed cataracts, etc.). She should be asked about previous falls and what caused them.
- Her past medical history should be recorded. She should be asked what medications she takes and consideration given as to whether these might cause her to fall, e.g. diuretics and sedatives. She must be asked about allergies.
- Her social history is vitally important. It must be decided if she will be able to cope at home. She should be asked what sort of home she lives in: flat (is there a lift to her floor?), house or bungalow; whether she lives alone and whether she has any help – who does her shopping, cleaning and cooking? Hand dominance should be established.

Examination

- The patient should be offered appropriate and adequate

analgesia before commencing the examination.

- If a medical reason for her fall is suspected then she should undergo a full physical examination, with particular attention paid to the cardiovascular (including lying and standing blood pressures) and neurological systems.
- Her wrist should be examined.
- The skin should be inspected, wounds might indicate a compound fracture.
- The radial pulse should identified, and the capillary refill of the fingers assessed.
- The nerves to the hand should be examined, in particular the median nerve.

9

Colles' fracture (2)

Some 3 months later you see the same woman in the fracture clinic. She has had her cast off for the last month and now complains of difficulty in holding a cup of tea. Examination of the wrist joint reveals that she has nearly normal flexion and extension of the wrist, and wasting of the thenar eminence. She also complains of tingling in the thumb.

1. What further examination would you perform?
2. What is the most likely diagnosis from the clinical findings?

Answer follows . . .

9

Colles' fracture (2)

Answer

1. A neurological examination of the hand is required. Inspection has already revealed wasting of the thenar eminence, and therefore it is likely that there will be weakness of these muscles. The ability to hold the index finger against the thumb will be reduced.

- **Median nerve** is tested as follows: motor function includes opposition (holding the thumb and little finger together), abduction (hold the patient's hand flat with the palm facing upwards and ask them to push their thumb upwards against your hand) and flexion (pull the thumb inwards against resistance). Touching the hand lightly with an orange-stick (never a sharp needle) demonstrates areas of reduced sensation.

- **Phalen's test** is performed by hyperflexing the wrist and asking whether there is an increase in the symptoms felt in the thumb.

- **Tinel's test** is performed by tapping on the median nerve and seeing if this increases symptoms in the thumb.

If these tests are normal, another cause of this patient's hand weakness should be considered (e.g. spinal lesion) and a full neurological examination performed.

2. The symptoms and signs indicate she has median nerve entrapment. This patient has developed a carpal tunnel syndrome as a complication of her fracture. Electromyography may be useful in doubtful cases.

10

Scaphoid fracture

You are working as an SHO in A&E when you see a man who fell off his bicycle on to his outstretched hand 1 day ago. He is complaining of a sore wrist. You notice he has swelling and tenderness in his anatomical snuffbox. There are no other injuries.

1. Examine this man's hand and describe the signs of a scaphoid fracture.
2. You request a radiograph of his scaphoid which the radiologist tells you is normal. How would you manage this case?

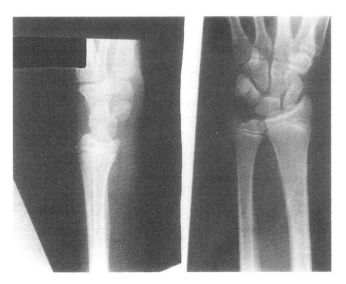

Figure 3.2

Scaphoid fracture

Answer

The important thing to remember is that the person sitting in front of you in the exam will be an actor, and so it is your job to act along too.

The actor will make the findings obvious (i.e. bony tenderness over the scaphoid), but you have to know how to look for it. Questions may be asked at the end, e.g. What are the complications?

1. Fullness and tenderness of the anatomical snuffbox (the hollow at the base of the thumb), pain on 'telescoping' the thumb (holding the thumb straight and pressing the thumb into the wrist) and pain on moving the thumb suggest a scaphoid fracture.
2. The initial radiograph of a scaphoid fracture is frequently normal. Further radiographs 14 days later may show a fracture after bony resorption has occurred. In the meantime, the wrist should be immobilised either in a splint or a plaster of Paris. Failure to do this may result in the development of avascular necrosis of the scaphoid.

4

Resuscitation

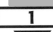

1

Management of the airway (basic)

Mrs Gordon, a 78-year-old smoker and a known emphysema patient, is admitted onto the respiratory ward as an inpatient. You are on night duty for the medical team covering the wards. You are called by the nurse to see Mrs Gordon because she is looking cyanosed and her saturations are only 76% despite receiving oxygen by mask. Please describe how you would respond to this call.

Answer follows . . .

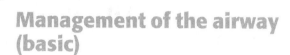

Management of the airway (basic)

Answer

Airway management is one of the simplest and yet most essential procedures that you will ever be asked to perform.

An obstructed airway can either be the cause of a patient losing consciousness, or may arise as a consequence of it. In either circumstance, the purpose of maintaining a patent airway is the same. In the conscious patient, airway obstruction will cause extreme distress and very quickly lead to a loss of consciousness. Airway obstruction may occur at any level from the mouth to the lungs. It may be that foreign matter is present in the airway – such as food, vomit or dentures – or it may be that the patient's own tongue and palate are occluding the airway, or that the airway is obstructed because it is swollen or oedematous. The patient may be in a coma, electrocuted or exposed to a noxious gas or chemicals. You **must** ensure your own safety before treating any patient (see the section on 'Basic Life Support' below).

Hypoxic brain injury occurs only **4** minutes after an airway is occluded. It is therefore essential that, irrespective of **any** other problems, the airway takes priority in your management of a patient.

Is the airway obstructed?

In every patient you ever meet, this should be the first

question you ask yourself. Of course, for the majority of your patients the answer will be 'No', but how do you recognise a patient with an obstructed airway?

One of the safest ways that is taught is the '**look**, **listen** and **feel**' approach.

Look

Is there any movement at the chest and/or abdomen? A 'seesaw' movement of the chest and abdomen is seen on respiratory effort in a patient with complete obstruction of the airway. Often this effort is extreme, even including the accessory muscles.

Listen

Can you hear air moving at the patient's mouth and nose? If you can hear breathing what does it sound like?

- **Silence**: This is possibly complete airway obstruction.
- **Inspiratory noises**, such as stridor: A high-pitched, harsh/creaking noise suggests upper airway obstruction.
- **Expiratory noises**, such as wheeze: A squeaking or puffing sound suggests lower airway obstruction.
- **Crowing**: This may suggest laryngeal spasm.
- **Snoring**: This may suggest the pharynx is partially occluded by the tongue.
- **Gurgling**: This may suggest the presence of semi-solid or liquid matter (such as vomitus or saliva) along the airway.

Feel

Feel for breath as the patient exhales.

Management

Having identified airway obstruction, management must be immediate.

Head tilt/chin lift/jaw thrust

The possibility of a neck injury must always be considered in traumatised patients and extra care is mandatory when protecting the airway.

In the neutral or flexed position, the tongue may lie in contact with the posterior wall of the pharynx and the epiglottis may occlude the laryngeal inlet. By tilting the head, the anterior neck muscles are stretched and these structures are pulled forwards. The head should not be tilted unless other techniques have failed. However, although it may be necessary to immobilise the neck completely, it is still possible to protect the airway using the following techniques.

Head tilt
(**Note:** If the patient has been fitted with a hard collar, perform a jaw thrust (see below) instead of a head tilt/chin lift.)
- Shout for help (or use your mobile phone to summon help).
- Turn the patient on her back and open her airway by performing a head tilt, i.e. place your hand over her forehead and gently tilt her head back. Keep your index finger and thumb of the same hand free to pinch the patient's nose for rescue breathing (see the section on 'Adult Basic Life Support' below).

Chin lift
Lifting the chin moves the mandible anteriorly, so amplifying the effects of the head tilt. The airway can be maintained with the head in this 'sniffing the morning air' position. If there is any suspicion of a neck injury then, with care, this manoeuvre can be performed without extending the neck at all.
- Open the patient's jaw and look inside her mouth for

any foreign bodies, e.g. loose dentures (**don't** use a finger to check). Only remove a foreign body if it is easy to see.
- With the patient supine, place your index and middle fingers under the mid-point of the mandible, and very gently lift it upwards, moving the chin anteriorly. With your thumb of the same hand, lightly grasp the lower lip and open the patient's mouth. Alternatively, the thumb may be placed inside the mouth behind the lower incisors and the chin lifted carefully.

Jaw thrust

With care, the mandible can be displaced anteriorly with no movement of the neck at all. This technique is particularly useful if a patient is being ventilated with a bag/mask device because it allows an excellent seal to be achieved while still maintaining the airway.
- Stand behind the patient's head and feel for the angles of her jaw.
- Place the index and middle fingers of both your hands behind the angles of the patient's jaw and apply steady upwards and forwards pressure.
- Use your thumb to open the jaw slightly by downward displacement of the chin.
- Check that the patient's breathing has improved – look, listen, feel.

However, if the patient does not improve:

- Look for other causes of obstruction.
- Remove foreign bodies/broken or dislodged dentures by performing a finger-sweep: using your right index finger, sweep the mouth cavity from left to right and gently ease out the foreign body. As far as possible, avoid doing this 'blind' as you may drive the foreign body distally towards the throat.
- If this fails, the next step is to consider more advanced techniques, using a Guedel oropharyngeal airway or a

nasopharyngeal airway (see below).

Definitive airways

These devices are designed to prevent the tongue falling backwards and obstructing the airway. However, a definitive airway must only be sited by a specifically trained individual – for example, an advanced life-support provider.

There are three definitive airways available:
- orotracheal tube
- nasotracheal tube
- surgical airway (e.g. tracheostomy or cricothyroidotomy).

Oropharyngeal (Guedel) airway

This is a small, plastic device which, when properly sized and inserted into the mouth, lifts the tongue away from the posterior wall of the pharynx. It does not, by itself, maintain the airway, and should be used with care in a semi-conscious patient as it may cause the patient to gag and vomit. Therefore, it is only tolerated in unconscious patients with no pharyngeal reflex, e.g. GCS < 10.

Inserting a Guedel airway

- You will need:
  - oxygen mask for spontaneous breathing
  - face mask (for artificial ventilation)
  - self-inflating bag (adult bags = 1500 ml) (reservoir bag can deliver up to 98% of oxygen)
  - a T-piece and open-ended bags
  - a flowmeter capable of delivering 15 litres of oxygen.
- Select an appropriate-sized Guedel airway: measure from the centre of the incisor teeth to the angle of the mandible by placing the Guedel airway concave side up into the patient's mouth.
- Use a chin lift (see above) to open the patient's airway,

taking care not to move her neck if a cervical trauma is suspected.

- Insert the tube concave side up until it reaches the junction between the hard and soft palates.
- Rotate through 180°, so the convex side is now up, and slide it back over the tongue (following the slope of the tongue). The flange should remain outside the mouth, distal to the incisors
- Re-check the patency of the airway.
- Consider a different size if in doubt.
- Place the oxygen mask over the airway tube if the patient's breathing is compromised (usually, oxygen or ventilation is always provided).
- Check that the patient's breathing, colour and oxygen saturation is improving.
  Note: An oropharyngeal tube may be unsuitable if the patient gags or strains. You should abandon the procedure and gently remove the tube along the curved dorsum of the tongue.

Nasopharyngeal airway

This is a long, thin plastic tube, which, when properly sized and inserted into one nostril, also lifts the tongue from the back of pharynx. Again, it does not, by itself, maintain the airway. This device must also be used with caution. Insertion may cause trauma and bleeding, which may further compromise the airway, and it must **never** be used in patients with a fracture of the base of the skull.

Consider fitting a nasopharyngeal airway if the patient is retching or has a gag reflex. It is often better tolerated than a Guedel airway.

Inserting a nasopharyngeal airway

- Select an airway of appropriate length and diameter. To obtain the appropriate length, hold the tube from the tip of the patient's nose to the tragus of her ear. An appropriate diameter tube is one that fits into the nostril without causing blanching; a rough guide to the tube diameter is to measure the tip of the patient's little finger.

- Lubricate the tube with K-Y jelly or a water-soluble lubricant, and insert a large safety-pin through the flange.
- Check the nostril for any septal deviation, then insert the tip and direct it posteriorly along the floor of the nose (rather than upwards).
- Rotate the tube gently as it passes the turbinates. A palpable 'give' denotes that the tube has passed the narrow area inside nose.
- Continue to pass the tube until the safety-pin rests on the nostril.
- Try the other nostril if there is difficulty inserting the tube, or use one of a smaller diameter (if a smaller tube is not available, a standard laryngeal tube can be cut to the correct length).
- Re-check the airway patency.
- Provide oxygen by mask, or by ventilation.

Questions and answers

Question: What are the complications of a longer nasopharyngeal tube?

Answer: An inappropriate size causes laryngospasm or mucosal trauma and can worsen airway obstruction.

Question: What are the contraindications of nasopharyngeal intubation?

Answer: Nasopharyngeal intubation is contraindicated in patients with an anterior basal skull fracture or significant haemorrhage from a friable nasal mucosa. There is a chance of bleeding in patients on anticoagulants.

Question: What precaution has to be taken for defibrillation during cardiopulmonary resuscitation (CPR)?

Answer: Oxygen is flammable. It should be switched off during defibrillation as a spark can cause fire.

Question: What saturation of oxygen is supplied with different masks?

Answer:
- A standard oxygen mask can deliver up to 50% of oxygen (only 10 litres of oxygen is recommended).
- A Venturi mask can deliver 24–60%.
- A mask with a reservoir bag can deliver up to 85% oxygen (with a 10–15 L oxygen supply).
- Self-inflating masks (need to hold the bag over the patient's mouth, with a leak) – connect to the oxygen supply, squeeze the bag, a one-way valve delivers high oxygen:
  - 45% oxygen (with an oxygen supply of 4–6 L)
  - 85% oxygen (with an oxygen supply of 10 L).

2

Oxygen therapy

Mr Jones is brought to A&E in a hypoxic state; the paramedics have given him oxygen. Please discuss oxygen therapy.

Answer

Oxygen is a drug. Like all other drugs, it has possible side-effects and needs to be prescribed at appropriate dosages.

Although oxygen is life saving in many instances, it is important to know how to handle it with care. This section reiterates many small safety factors that PLAB candidates should be aware of, particularly when treating the hypoxic patient.

Measurement

Arterial oxygen saturation (SaO_2)

The simplest way to measure the amount of oxygen circulating in the body is to use simple pulse oximetry (arterial oxygen saturation, SaO_2); normal ranges lie between 95 and 100%. However, it is important to note that values are likely to be inaccurate in patients with poorly perfused extremities and those suffering from carbon monoxide poisoning. In such cases, and where oxygen saturation readings are less than 93%, it may be worthwhile to consider requesting arterial blood gas measurements, which give a more accurate assessment of oxygen saturation.

Arterial blood gas (ABG)

An ABG sample can give a rapid and detailed picture of a

patient's acid–base balance. Generally, (but not exclusively) the radial artery is used, a heparinised syringe is essential and the sample should be analysed as quickly as possible.

Normal values:
- pH – 7.35–7.45
- $p(O_2)$ – 10–13 kPa (75–100 mmHg)
- $p(CO_2)$ – 4.8–6.1 kPa (36–46 mmHg)
- HCO_3 – 22–26 mmol/L
- Base excess ± 2

Administration

For a conscious patient who is unlikely to tolerate any airway adjuncts (see Management of the airway (basic)), there are three forms of equipment at your disposal.

- **Nasal cannulas:** These supply a maximum of 28% oxygen and are generally less claustrophobic than oxygen masks; however, make sure your patient is not mouth-breathing as this will result in the cannula being far less effective.
- **Venturi mask:** This supplies a maximum of about 60% oxygen.
- **Non-rebreather mask:** Such a mask will supply a maximum of about 85% oxygen and is probably your first choice in an unwell, but conscious, patient (depending, of course, upon the individual patient).

Humidified oxygen

This is given when oxygen is to be used in the longer term rather than for immediate therapy. It can reach a maximum of about 80%, is less drying than standard oxygen, is kinder generally and safer in asthmatic patients in particular.

Nebulised oxygen

Nebulised oxygen, or oxygen going through with a

nebuliser, can usually reach a maximum of about 35%. If higher flow rates are required then change back as soon as the nebuliser is complete.

Delivery

Ideally, oxygen should be specifically prescribed for each patient to avoid errors in management.

Paramedics will generally bring most patients into A&E on high-flow oxygen, regardless of the initial complaint. It is your job to assess whether or not the level of administration needs to be altered, and in certain cases it is crucial to do this as soon as possible.

As a rule, patients should be given the lowest inspired oxygen concentrations compatible with adequate arterial oxygenation.

A prime example is in patients with COPD (chronic obstructive pulmonary disease). Such patients present with a type II respiratory failure, where there is both hypoxaemia and hypercapnia (i.e. they 'retain' carbon dioxide). Normally the major stimulant to the respiratory centre is carbon dioxide. In patients with COPD the chronically elevated levels of carbon dioxide result in hypoxaemia becoming the major drive to breathe. In effect, it is important to correct the hypercapnia rather than focusing on the hypoxaemia. Therefore, *you must **never** give more than 2 L or 24% oxygen to a patient with COPD.*

Domiciliary oxygen

Many patients are candidates for home oxygen therapy.

Depending upon individual requirements, some patients require prn oxygen at home. The provision of domiciliary oxygen cylinders can be arranged by local GP practices; others need larger amounts of oxygen (see below). The amount of oxygen required is based on arterial blood gas findings on air and on various flow rates of oxygen.

Long-term oxygen therapy (LTOT) is often required by patients with end-stage COPD, or those with an oxygen reading of less than 7.3 kPa on air. LTOT involves the continual delivery of oxygen over 15 hours of the day, every day. (Note that LTOT has not been proven to decrease morbidity or mortality in patients with pulmonary fibrosis.)

For people who require large amounts of oxygen, the number of cylinders required may be inappropriate. Therefore an 'oxygen concentrator' can be requested via the local GP practice, which cuts down on the number of individual cylinders needed and is more convenient.

Ventilation

Remember that oxygen is used in measures of respiratory support, and it is a good idea to be aware of some of the different measures of ventilation. However, it is unlikely you will be asked about these as a part of the PLAB exam.

WARNING!
A quick reminder, oxygen is flammable, **always** remove the oxygen source during defibrillation!

Discussion

Possible questions
1. A known COPD patient presents to you with an exacerbation of his condition. What flow rate of oxygen would you like to start the patient on and why?
2. An elderly lady in LVF presents to you with SOB. How would you assess her level of hypoxia and when would an arterial blood gas measurement be warranted?
3. A young, asthmatic girl presents with a severe wheeze and dry cough, her laboured breathing is making her tired. What type of oxygen might it be wise to request?

3

Basic life support (adult)

You are on night duty attending to a confused patient on the elderly care ward when you suddenly hear a thud in the next cubicle. You draw back the curtain to see an elderly man lying on the floor, he appears to be unconscious. There are no other staff in the immediate vicinity, how would you respond?

Answer follows . . .

3

Basic life support (adult)

Answer

For the purpose of basic life support (BLS), the Resuscitation Council (UK) describes an 'adult' as any person over the age of 8 years.

The purpose of basic life support, which may either take place inside or outside a hospital environment, is to ensure that the patient's vital organs continue to receive oxygenated blood. The process incorporates assessment of the patient and maintenance of adequate ventilation and circulation until the underlying problem can be addressed.

Remember, always use a SAFE approach: Shout, Approach, Free, Evaluate.

SAFE

S – Shout for help

Shout '**Help**'. If you have a mobile phone, use it to call for help. You must not leave the patient at this time.

A – Approach with care

Look for signs of danger that may harm **you**. Has the patient been electrocuted or exposed to hazardous chemicals? (**Remember**: avoid assisted ventilation without a mask since, for example, organophosphates are easily absorbed through the skin and can be present in saliva and air droplets, or the patient may have a virus infection.) Is there busy traffic or falling masonry, etc?

Approach the patient only when dangers have been addressed (two emergencies are **not** better than one!)

F – Free from danger

If the patient is in a dangerous position then, if possible, move them to a place of safety. For example, when approaching the patient you would make sure that a train is not coming; then, without endangering yourself, you would free them from danger by moving them away from the tracks.

E – Evaluate 'ABC' (Airway **– B**reathing **– C**irculation)

Is the patient responsive? Speaking loudly and clearly, ask: 'Are you alright?'. Gently shake the patient by the shoulder as you do this. If the patient responds:
- Leave him in that position and check for signs of injury.
- At regular intervals, re-check the patient and seek help.

Management

Follow the ABC rule.

Airway

If the patient does not respond during your evaluation:
- Shout for help (or use your mobile phone to call for help).
- If you can assess the patient in the position you find them, do so; if not, then carefully turn them onto their back, look for a foreign body in their mouth and open their airway using the techniques described in the 'Management of the airway' section above.

Breathing

While continuing to protect the airway, look, listen and feel

for breathing (this must take no more than 10 seconds):
- **look** for chest movements
- **listen** for breath sounds at the patient's mouth
- **feel** for air from the patient's mouth on your cheek.

If the patient breathes:
- Place them in the recovery position and seek help.

If the patient is not breathing (or making ineffective attempts to breathe):
- Call for help on a mobile phone. If one isn't available, send someone for help.
- If you are alone and cannot summon help, when should you go for help?:
  - In an adult where the cause of unconsciousness is likely to be cardiac, you should leave the patient and get help at once.
  - In an adult where the cause of unconsciousness is likely to be respiratory (causes of which include drowning, choking, intoxication or trauma), you should perform resuscitation (see below) for 1 minute and then summon help.
- At the earliest opportunity, give **two** 'slow, effective rescue breaths' as follows:
  - Ensure a patent airway (head tilt/chin lift): pinch the nostrils shut while supporting the forehead with the palm of the same hand, and with your other hand gently open the patient's mouth (while keeping the airway patent).
  - Next, take a deep breath to fill your own lungs and place your lips around the patient's mouth, ensuring a good seal. (A deep breath will increase the oxygenation of your exhaled air.)
  - Steadily exhale and watch the patient's chest rise. This will take around 2 s.
  - Keeping the airway patent, move your head away from the patient. Watch the chest fall as the patient exhales.
  - Take another deep breath and repeat this process. It is

important that two effective breaths are given. The Resuscitation Council Guidelines allow for five attempts to make two effective rescue breaths.

Circulation

After **two** effective breaths, or after a **total of five** attempts, move on to assess the circulation:

- Feel for a carotid pulse by placing two fingers gently to the side of the Adam's apple (cricoid cartilage), but:
  - **do not** feel for longer than 10 s
  - **never** feel for a pulse on both sides at the same time.
- If you detect a pulse – continue rescue breaths until the patient starts breathing by himself.
- Every 10 breaths (approximately every 60 s), recheck for a pulse as above.
- If you do not detect a pulse (or if you are not sure) – start chest compressions.

Chest compressions

Find the correct position for chest compressions as follows:

- Using the middle finger of your hand nearest to the patient's feet, feel along the costal margin until you reach the xiphoid process.
- Then place the heel of your other hand next to the index finger. This position should be the middle of the lower half of the sternum.
- Keeping the heel of your hand in this position, release the two fingers on the lower sternum and place the heel of this hand on top of the other and interlock the fingers.
- Take care not to press on the patient's abdomen or xiphisternum.
- For each chest compression, position yourself vertically above the patient and firmly press the sternum down 4–5 cm while keeping your arms straight. When you release the pressure take care not to lose contact, but allow the sternum to rise again ready for the next compression.

- Chest compressions should be performed at a rate of 100 per minute.
- After 15 compressions, perform two more effective breaths and continue with this ratio of 15:2.

When should you stop?

- You should only stop to reassess the patient if they move or breathe without help.
- Continue with your resuscitation (compressions and effective breaths) until support arrives.

4

Basic life support (paediatric)

You are called to a 6-year-old child who appears to be unconscious. Describe what you would do.

Answer follows . . .

4

Basic life support (paediatric)

Answer

In general, the principles of paediatric BLS are the same as for adults; however, the technique varies with the child's age. For the purposes of BLS, children under 1 year of age are classed as infants and those between 1 and 8 years as small children; children over 8 years of age are treated as adults.

Since anoxia is the main cause of cardiac arrest in those under 8 years of age, airway management takes precedence over defibrillation. With BLS you can give adequate support to vital functions, but, as this is the foundation of advanced life support, the correct technique is important.

Remember, always use the same SAFE approach as for adult BLS: **S**hout; **A**pproach; **F**ree; **E**valuate.

SAFE

S – Shout for help
See the BLS (adult) section above.

A – Approach with care
See the BLS (adult) section above.

F – Free from danger
See the BLS (adult) section above.

E – Evaluate 'ABC' (Airway – **B**reathing – **C**irculation)
Stand on the child's right side (if you are right-handed).
Where there is a risk of injury, protect the child's neck by
placing one hand firmly on his/her forehead. Ask clearly
and loudly, 'Are you all right?' If there is no response,
shake the child gently by the shoulder – a conscious child
may respond by answering, making a sound or opening
their eyes.

Management
Follow the ABC rule: airway, breathing, circulation.

Airway

Is there an obvious airway obstruction?
- Look inside the child's mouth to see if there is an
  obvious foreign body obstructing his/her airway; and,
  providing you can do so easily, remove it.
  *Is the child fully conscious but having difficulty in
  breathing?*
- Take the child to hospital immediately.
  *Is the child in a comfortable position for breathing, e.g.
  sitting on the mother's lap, or lying in bed?*
- Then **do not** disturb, leave him in that position.

Breathing

If the child is not breathing:
- Use the **head tilt** to open the airway by placing your
  palm over the child's forehead then tilting their head
  back slightly; for:
  - **infants**: tilt their head to neutral
  - **child**: tilt their head to the sniffing position.
- Perform **chin lift** by placing two fingers of your other
  hand under the child's chin and gently tilting it upwards.
  Make sure this doesn't close the child's mouth. Keep the
  lips open with your thumb if required.

- Look, listen, feel (bring your cheek over the child's face, your ear over the child's nose and look across to his/her chest for no longer than 10 seconds):
  - **look** for chest and abdominal movements for breathing
  - **listen** for breaths and sounds
  - **feel** for exhaled air from breathing.
- If you can not do a head tilt/chin lift, or it is contraindicated (trauma), use the **jaw thrust** method to open the airway as follows:
  - Place two or three fingers behind the angle of the jaw on both sides and lift the jaw upwards (resting both your elbows on the same surface as child's head may help to steady your hands), then tilt the child's head slightly.
- Look, listen and feel as before.
- If spontaneous breathing has not started with 10 seconds perform initial rescue breathing (aim for at least **two** effective breaths) as follows:
  - Take a deep breath, seal the child's mouth, or mouth and nose, and slowly give a rescue breath for 1–1.5 s. If you only seal the child's mouth, pinch his/her nose closed with your thumb and index fingers while tilting the child's head with your other hand. (Breathing in deeply increases the oxygenation of your exhaled air.)
  - Check for chest rise as you exhale. Don't blow too hard or too fast. Blowing softly at a low pressure reduces gastric distension.
- Check the child's pulse.
- Only when rescue breathing is successful, go on to the circulation.

Circulation

- Check the central pulse for 10 s – use the brachial artery in infants or the carotid pulse in small children.
- If a pulse is present (of adequate volume and rate

sufficient to maintain circulation) – continue exhaled air ventilation until spontaneous breathing is restored.

- If there is no pulse after 10 s or only a slow pulse (less that 60 beats/min), or there is no sign of circulation, place the child, on his back, on a flat, hard surface and start CPR as follows (rate of compression for all ages – 100/min):

  Under 1 year of age:
  - **position**: one finger-breadth below an imaginary line joining both nipples
  - **depth**: one-third of the infant's chest
  - **technique**: use two fingers to compress the chest
  - **rate**: 5 compressions to 1 ventilation

  or
  - use the 'hand-circling technique' (but only if two rescuers are available), i.e.: encircle, or partly encircle, the baby's chest with both your hands, placing both thumbs in the correct position as described above.

  Small children:
  - **position**: one finger-breadth above the xiphisternum
  - **technique**: use the heel of one hand
  - **rate**: 5 compressions to 1 ventilation.

  Larger children:
  - **position**: two finger-breadths above the xiphisternum
  - **technique**: use the heels of both hands
  - **rate**: 15 compressions to 2 ventilations.

- If there is no improvement after **1 minute** of CPR, contact the emergency services (shout or use your mobile phone to call for help, you shouldn't leave the patient).

Questions and answers

Question: Why is breathing more important?

Answer: Because anoxia is the main cause of cardiac arrest in children under 8 years of age.

Question: What does it mean if the chest doesn't rise

during mouth-to-mouth resuscitation?

Answer: The airway is not clear.

Question: What is the main cause of ventilation or CPR failure?

Answer: Failed technique.

Question: How can you improve the ventilation technique?

Answer: Correct the head tilt/chin lift, and try again. Otherwise, try the jaw thrust method.

Question: Why should you give five rescue breaths?

Answer: The Resuscitation Council Guidelines allow for five attempts to make two effective rescue breaths; and, depending on the circumstances, at least two will be effective.

Question: Why is feeling for the carotid pulse not recommended in infants?

Answer: Babies have short and fat necks.

Question: What other signs tell you there is no circulation?

Answer:
- no pulse
- inadequate volume or rate (very thin), or arrhythmia (bradycardia, tachycardia)
- no breath or cough when a rescue breath is given
- no spontaneous movement.

Question: What other pulse can be checked in infants?

Answer: The brachial or femoral pulse.

Question: Why are two rescuers required for the hand-encircling CPR technique?

Answer: If only one person is available then the time taken to re-position the airway and give ventilation may delay performing compressions.

Question: Is there a recovery position for infants?

Answer: No satisfactory recovery position has yet been identified. However, the rescuer should check that the airway is being maintained, observe the infant until help arrives and ensure the baby is not lying on pressure points.

Question: What is the problem for a solo rescuer?

Answer: Maintaining a full cycle of compression and efficiency and adequacy of CPR, calling for help, etc. Readjusting the airway or re-establishing the correct method of compression will decrease the number of CPR cycles that can be given by a solo rescuer.

Question: When do you stop?

Answer: You don't stop CPR until the child moves or takes a breath.

Question: Do you need to check your position for each compression cycle?

Answer: Providing the position was correct at the start, it should not be measured after each ventilation; doing so will seriously compromise the effectiveness of CPR.

5

Neonatal resuscitation

Unless you are trained in neonatal resuscitation, always ask the nurse or midwife to page the senior paediatrician or the duty anaesthetist, and ask the midwife to stand by the phone while you return to the baby.

Method

- Start the clock, or check the time (you will be working against time).
- Dry the baby, wrap him in a blanket and keep him warm.

Assessment

Assess the baby for:
- **Colour**:
  - a pink baby, with a fast (> 100 beats/min) heart rate is usually a healthy baby
  - a blue baby with a slow heart rate (60 beats/min or less), with inadequate breathing needs gentle stimulation
  - a blue or white, apnoeic baby, with a very slow heart rate (< 60 beats/min), or absent heart rate, is a very poorly baby.
- **Respiration** – rate and quality?
- **Heart rate** – fast, slow, absent?
- **Tone** – unconscious, apnoiec babies are floppy

Management

The resuscitation procedure remains the same as always, namely ABC (airway, breathing and circulation), with the use of medication if required.

Airway

- Hold the baby's head in a neutral position (e.g. place a folded towel under its neck and shoulders). Be careful, too much neck extension or flexion may collapse the baby's airway.
- If the baby does not breathe – use a jaw thrust to open the baby's airway, then suck the nares and oropharynx with a soft-suction catheter, this may start respiration. Avoid deep throat suction as this may cause bradycardia or laryngospasm.

Breathing

- If the baby does not breathe – give five inflation breaths (2–3 min each).
- Reassess the baby for visible chest movements or an increase in its heart rate.
- No response – check head position again, check jaw thrust, then give another five inflation breaths.
- Reassess the baby for visible chest movements or an increase in heart rate.
- Still no response – ask for help. Tell the examiner you need help with the baby's airway and with giving inflation breaths.
- Open the baby's mouth, use a torch to visibly inspect the oropharynx and repeat the inflation breaths.
- Now you need to insert an oropharyngeal airway and repeat the inflationary breaths.
- Select the correct-sized Guedel airway tube by measuring the distance from the angle of the baby's mouth to the angle of its jaw.
- Gently open the baby's mouth, point the tip of the airway tube upwards towards the hard palate, then gently insert it without force, finally rotate the tip to point downwards, so the airway tube lies over the dorsum of the tongue.
- Consider intubation (tell the examiner you need the help

of a senior or paediatric anaesthetist to insert the airway).

- Again check response: chest movement or an increase in heart rate.
- When the chest is moving continue to give ventilation breaths if there is no spontaneous breathing.

Circulation

- Check the baby's heart rate – if there is no heart beat, or it is slow (60 beats/min or less) and not rising, start chest compressions.
- Check chest expansion, if there is no movement re-check the airway, then start cycles of **three** chest compressions to **one** breath for 30 s.
- Reassess:
  - if improving – stop chest compressions
  - if not breathing – continue ventilation
  - if the heart rate is still slow – continue ventilation and chest compressions.
- Tell the examiner you wish to gain venous or intraosseous access and to start medication.

Questions and answers

Question: What is the significance of meconium aspiration, and how would you deal with it?

Answer: Some staining is common. Aspiration, however, is rare. I would clear the baby's mouth, nose and perineum of meconium. If unresponsive, greater clearance with a wide-bore suction tube, using a laryngoscope to visualise the oropharynx, may be required. If still unresponsive, I would clear the trachea through the endotracheal tube.

Question: What pressure should be used for suction?

Answer: It should not exceed 100 mmHg (9.8 kPa).

Question: What is an inflation breath and how would you give them?

Answer: The first five breaths are inflation breaths, each lasting 2–3 s, and are delivered using high-flow oxygen, a pressure-limiting device and a mask. I would use a transparent, circular, soft mask that could cover the baby's mouth and nose.

Question: If a baby mask was unavailable what would you do?

Answer: I would use a 500-ml self-inflating bag fitted with a blow-off valve, set at 30–40 cm/min.

Question: Why may the chest not expand immediately after giving inflation breaths?

Answer: The chest may not move for the first 1–3 breaths because fluid is being displaced.

Question: Can you say the baby is inhaling if you hear breath sounds on auscultation and how would you check?

Answer: Not for first few breaths, as fluid-filled lungs can transmit sound. I would assess whether the baby is inhaling by checking its chest expansion.

Question: At what rate should a baby be ventilated?

Answer: 30–40 cm/min.

Question: When do you need to start CPR?

Answer: When heart rate is 60 beats/min or below, and the chest is expanding.

Question: Describe how do you start CPR?

Answer: Encircle the baby's chest with both hands, apposing thumbs on the sternum, just below the internipple line. Compress briskly to one-third of its depth, give three compressions for each chest inflation.

Question: Which comes first, the heart or the lungs, and why?

Answer: The lungs. ABC is the resuscitation sequence. Unless the blood is oxygenated, the heart will not recover.

Question: When may drug therapy be given in neonatal resuscitation?

Answer: Only after adequate resuscitation attempts have been made, especially to establish a patent airway and breathing.

Question: What vein is used to give drugs?

Answer: The umbilical vein.

Question: Discuss the drugs usually given in neonatal resuscitation.

Answer:
- Adrenaline – 10 μg/kg of 1:10,000 adrenaline. Give repeat doses of 10–30 μg/kg every 3–5 min.
- Bicarbonate solution – 1 mmol/kg (2 ml/kg of a 4.2% solution).
- Dextrose (glucose) – 5 ml/kg of 10% dextrose (glucose), followed by 100 ml/kg per day of 10% dextrose (glucose). (Blood glucose sticks are unreliable for readings <5 mmol/L).
- Fluid – occasional – 10 ml/kg (in haemorrhage or septicaemia).
- Naloxone – 10 μg/kg (effect lasts for 20 min).

Suturing

Please put two simple stitches into the cut.

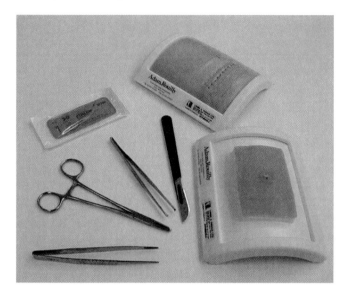

Figure 5.1

Answer follows . . .

1

Suturing

Answer

This is the usual instruction for this station and the stitches will be into simulated skin (manikin). It is a skill that should be practised beforehand. If you have done a lot of suturing, use the method you find the most comfortable; however, for the purposes of the exam, it is preferable to stitch by hand.

Steps (this is an aseptic technique)

1. Tell the examiner you would introduce yourself to the patient. Explain that this cut will need stitches to close it adequately. You will put in a local anaesthetic to numb the area; the injection will feel like a sharp scratch followed by a stinging sensation, but it will numb soon after. Say you would obtain the patient's permission to proceed.

2. Select your equipment – your mainstay of equipment will be toothed forceps, needle-holding forceps and scissors. You can have an assistant, ask them to open the outer (non-sterile) packaging of the suture kit. Wash your hands during this time.

3. Ask your assistant to open the outer packaging of the sterile gloves, put on your gloves and open up the suture kit.

4. Ask your assistant to pour sterile water into the available tray, then drop some 4–0 ethylon (this is nylon, which is a non-absorbable monofilament suture material) on to the sterile field.

5. With your assistant, double-check the label on the ampoule. Draw up 10 ml of 1% lidocaine (lignocaine) into a 10 ml syringe. Discard the needle used for drawing up (into a sharps bin, **make sure this is nearby**) and replace with a new (orange) needle.

6. Clean the skin with an alcohol wipe.

7. Infiltrate around the wound with the local anaesthetic, forewarning the patient of a sharp scratch. Always draw back on the syringe before injecting (looking out for a flashback to avoid injecting lidocaine intravenously).

8. Wait for the local anaesthetic to start working (5–10 min) and check for an allergic reaction.

9. Check the anaesthetic has taken effect by pinching the skin with toothed forceps.

10. Place two stitches, bisecting the wound in half and then bisecting again (equidistant).

11. Knot three times over each stitch.

12. Dispose of all sharps adequately into the nearby sharps bin.

13. Tell the patient that the stitches will have to come out in about a week, and to make an appointment for this with their GP. If they need a painkiller then simple paracetamol should be fine, which can be obtained over the counter.

14. Ask your assistant for a dressing and place it over the cut.

15. Thank the patient and assistant.

Discussion

Lidocaine (lignocaine)

Lidocaine is most frequently used as a local anaesthetic, 20 ml of 1% lidocaine can safely be used for an adult.

Given intravenously, lidocaine can cause arrhythmias and convulsions.

Adrenaline (epinephrine)

Adrenaline may be used, which may also help to minimise

bleeding. It is available in combination with lidocaine, e.g. 1:200,000 adrenaline with 2% lidocaine. However, the use of adrenaline is contraindicated in end-artery organs, such as fingers/toes, tip of the nose, penis and ear lobes because it may result in ischaemic necrosis.

Antibiotic cover and immunisation

The patient's tetanus immunisation status should be sought if the history suggests a particularly dirty wound. Booster doses can be given every 10 years.

If the patient is diabetic with poor control, it may be wise to suggest a 1-week course of flucloxacillin cover (but check for penicillin allergy first).

2

Bladder catheterisation

Please insert a catheter into this patient's bladder. He has no known history of prostatic enlargement or malignancy.

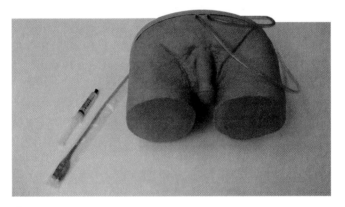

Figure 5.2

Answer follows . . .

2

Bladder catheterisation

Answer

There are many indications for urethral catheterisation, including urinary retention, accurate fluid balance, in certain pre-operative patients, etc. A manikin will be used for this station.

Remember that you should ask for a chaperone (preferably male) to be present at this station.

Steps (this is an aseptic technique)

1. Tell the examiner you would introduce yourself to the patient and explain that a plastic tube will have to be inserted into his 'water works'. This will make all the water stored in his bladder (the sack in the body containing urine) drain out freely, and will make him feel more comfortable. Mention that a local anaesthetic jelly will be used, and, although it should not hurt, he should say if he feels pain.

2. Select your equipment: catheter (go for the smallest 12F–14F), lidocaine (lignocaine) jelly, sterile gloves, 10 ml syringe pre-filled with 10 ml of water, catheter bag, sterile water or normal saline, cotton-wool balls, waste bag, sterile field, gauze pads.

3. As you wash your hands and put on your sterile gloves, ask your assistant (usually available at this station) to open the outer packaging of the pieces of equipment and to drop the items onto a sterile work surface.

4. Cut or tear a hole in the centre of the sterile field, and spread it over the patient's body so that his penis is visible through the hole.

5. The principle throughout the procedure is 'non-dominant hand dirty, dominant hand clean'. So, using your non-dominant hand, hold the penis upright and clean around the prepuce using cotton-wool and sterile water. Clean back from the meatus (to keep bacteria away from the orifice). Retract the foreskin to clean the glans.

6. Lidocaine (lignocaine) jelly can now be instilled through the urethral opening. While still holding the penis upright, allow 5–10 minutes for the anaesthetic to take effect. Mention you would generally wait this long and then carry on.

7. Now select the catheter, this will still be wrapped in its inner sterile bag. Tear along the perforations and remove the catheter tip, keeping the rest of the catheter in the bag.

8. Slowly insert the catheter – it should go in smoothly – until you reach the hilt, or until urine starts to pass through the catheter into the bag (indicating the catheter is in the bladder).

9. Inflate the balloon with the 10 ml of water in the pre-filled syringe. Ensure that this does not cause any pain before proceeding to the next stage.

10. Attach the catheter drainage bag to the end of the catheter.

11. Place the used items into the waste bag for correct disposal.

12. Mention that if a foreskin had been present then now would be the time to reduce it to avoid the development of a paraphimosis.

13. Mention you would like the nurses to document the residual volume.

14. Thank the patient and the assistant.

Discussion

Catheter not passing

This is generally due to a smooth muscle spasm, in which case you should stop the procedure and wait until the spasm passes before continuing.

If prostate enlargement is suspected (particularly malignant) and you are unable to continue passing the catheter beyond a certain point, ask a urologist for a specialist opinion.

Contraindications to catheterisation

- High-riding prostate (after pelvic trauma)
- Prostatic malignancy (relative contraindication)
- Urethral injury/fistula.

Anatomy

The male urethra is sigmoid-shaped with two kinks, and can be up to 18 cm long. For this reason it is important to hold the penis upright, 90 degrees to the supine body – this straightens the urethra, making the passage of a catheter smoother and less painful.

Anaesthetic

The lidocaine jelly has two functions: a local anaesthetic action, which becomes effective after about 5 minutes; and lubrication. Therefore some of the jelly can also be applied to the catheter tip. The patient can expect to feel uncomfortable, but it should not be too painful. However, if this is the case you should stop and seek help as urethral damage may otherwise occur.

Catheter

Foley catheters are used; 12–16 French (F) gauge will be available, go for a smaller one (the larger the gauge, the larger the catheter diameter). Long-term catheters are available that can stay in place for up to a month. Short-term catheters should be checked every few days.

Complications

- Infection and trauma are the two greatest complications.
- Torrential haemorrhage may occur in a patient with prostatic malignancy.

Cervical smear

Please perform a speculum examination on the manikin and take a cervical smear.

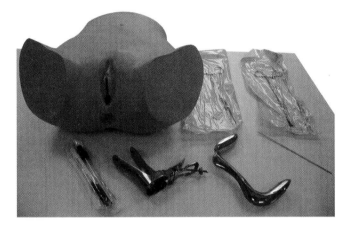

Figure 5.3

Answer follows . . .

3

Cervical smear

Answer

This is the usual instruction for this station. However, if a discharge is mentioned, you should take swabs to be taken (see Chapter 2, Vaginal discharge) – after speculum insertion.

Remember to ask for a chaperone (preferably female).

Steps

1. Tell the examiner you would introduce yourself to the patient. Explain that a speculum, a metal object to open the parts, will be inserted and then a sample of cells taken from the neck of her womb (the cervix). This sample will then be sent for analysis. Say that you would obtain the patient's permission to proceed.

2. Ask the woman (via examiner) to go behind the curtain and undress from the waist down, then lay on the couch with her feet together and her knees flopped apart. She may drape a towel over her thighs.

3. During this time start gathering your equipment together: gloves, a metal bivalve self-retaining Cusco's speculum in its sterile bag, lubricating jelly, Ayre's wooden spatula, tissues, Cytofix, clean glass slide, pencil, lab. request forms and plastic specimen bags.

4. Write the patient's name, hospital number, date and time of the specimen on the slide in pencil (the fixative makes ink disappear).

5. Adjust your light source and put on your gloves.
6. If you are a not a gynaecologist, familiarise yourself with a Cusco's speculum, it is self-retaining and this mechanism should be practised. Ask to warm the speculum in warm running water (metal can feel very cold, and very uncomfortable, for the patient!).
7. Lubricate the speculum with K-Y jelly.
8. Inspect the labia.
9. Open the labia using your non-dominant hand.
10. Introduce the speculum vertically in line with the labia, then turn it through 90°.
11. Now open up the speculum until you can see the cervix on the manikin. Lock the speculum into place.
12. Select the Ayre's spatula, you are aiming for the squamocolumnar junction, make a turn through 240°.
13. Spread the sample evenly over the whole slide and spray evenly with Cytofix. (Make sure you smear the sample on the labelled side!)
14. Unlock the speculum and gently remove it as it was inserted; it is important to do this slowly to avoid nipping the walls of the vagina.
15. Thank the patient, offer her tissues to wipe herself down. Say that she may now get dressed. Tell her she will get the results in about 2 weeks time through the post, and that any further queries should be put to her GP.
16. Label the smear form.

Discussion

Cytofix

Cytofix is a trade name for the fixative. It consists of 50% alcohol and 50% ether.

Before taking a smear

Ensure the patient:

- is not menstruating
- has not used a lubricant or spermicide in the last 24 hours.

If there is a discharge

- If an ulcer is present, it is important to take a swab from the base of the ulcer.
- If a chlamydial infection is suspected, take a high vaginal swab and a swab of the cervix.
- A vaginal swab is taken from the posterior fornix.
- Send the swabs for microscopy and for culture and sensitivity testing.

Equipment

- All sorts of different spatulas and speculums may be available in the exam., stick to what you know.
- The speculum itself has a metal arm with a disc on the end, this can be slotted through a metal flap with holes and screwed into place, therefore making it self-retaining.

4

Fundoscopy

Mr Helkios, an unwell man, has a past history of ischaemic heart disease, diabetes and hypertension. He presents to you with headache and blurred vision. Please perform a fundoscopic examination and describe your findings.

Answer follows . . .

4

Fundoscopy

Answer

Fundoscopy is the procedure used to visualise the retina (or 'the back of the eye') – and employs an ophthalmoscope.

A list of some of the abnormalities you may be able to identify through fundoscopy is given below; however, the following are the most important for the PLAB exam:
- diabetic retinopathy
- hypertensive retinopathy.

Steps

1. Introduce yourself to the patient/examiner (as appropriate).
2. Explain that you are about to examine the back of the eye, that this involves a bright light and may be a little uncomfortable, but it should not hurt.
3. Ensure the patient has understood, and obtain his permission to proceed.
4. Ideally, darken the room, and find a spot on which the patient can focus.
5. Stand back, place the ophthalmoscope to your right eye and focus it until you can see clearly. Next look for a red reflex in the patient's right eye (indicates a clear medium).
6. Follow the red reflex; then, getting closer to the eye, examine the lens for any opacity (cataract).

7. Visualise the retina for any abnormalities (discussed below). You may need to refocus the ophthalmoscope to adjust for the patient's eye.

8. Repeat the examination on the left eye (remember your left eye examines the patient's left eye).

9. Thank the patient/examiner for their co-operation (as appropriate).

10. Turn to the examiner and express your findings.

Tip: It's a good idea to place one hand on the patient's forehead to steady yourself – obtain the patient's permission first.

Discussion

You may be shown slides of various retinal pathology.

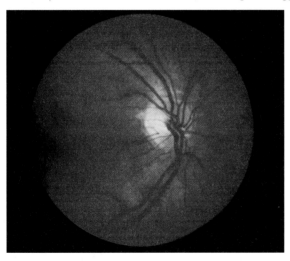

Figure 5.4 Example of normal retina.

Causes of retinal haemorrhages
- Diabetes mellitus:
  - Grade 1 – background retinopathy: this includes 'dot and blot' haemorrhages, sometimes 'hard exudates'

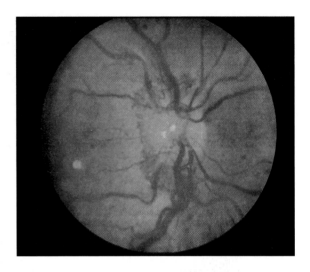

Figure 5.5 Example of diabetic retinal changes.

- ○ Grade 2 – pre-proliferative retinopathy: this may show 'cotton-wool' exudates
- ○ Grade 3 – proliferative retinopathy: this is neovascularisation, look for the growth of new fragile vessels; this condition requires urgent referral; treatment is by laser photocoagulation
- ○ Grade 4 – diabetic maculopathy: exudates appear within a disc width of the macula; this is common in type 2 diabetes and also requires laser therapy
- Hypertensive retinopathy:
  - ○ Grade 1 – tortuous vessels and 'silver wiring'
  - ○ Grade 2 – arteriovenous 'nipping'
  - ○ Grade 3 – flame-shaped haemorrhages and cotton-wool spots
  - ○ Grade 4 – papilloedema
- Trauma
- Central retinal vein occlusion (CRVO)
- Central retinal artery occlusion (CRAO – after 48 hours of occlusion)
- Sickle-cell disease.

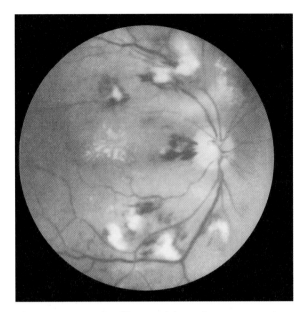

Figure 5.6 Example of hypertensive retina.

Causes of papilloedema (swelling of the disc):

- Increased intracranial pressure (e.g. sub-arachnoid haemorrhage, space-occupying lesion)
- Cerebral oedema
- Malignant hypertension
- Papillitis
- Pseudopapilloedema.

Causes of optic atrophy (pallor of the disc):

- Glaucoma
- Ischaemic optic atrophy
- Leber's optic atrophy
- Toxic methanol poisoning
- Tumours, e.g. craniopharyngioma.

5

Lung function tests (peak flow and spirometry)

Please discuss basic lung function tests.

Answer follows . . .

5

Lung function tests (peak flow and spirometry)

Answer

At the end of the respiratory examination, you may be asked about basic lung function tests. For a 5-minute OSCE you are not expected to go into detail, but it is important to be aware of some common types of tests, techniques and their uses.

Peak expiratory flow rate

This is a measure of lung function. Or more correctly, the maximum velocity with which a patient can blow air out of their lungs, measured in litres per minute.

The expected rate depends upon a number of variables, including age, sex, height and time of day.

Predicted charts are available, calculated according to height, sex and age. Average values range from:
- 400–650 L/min in males
- 300–500 L/min in females.

Instructions to the patient

- Ask the patient to stand (preferable) or sit upright.
- Hold the peak flow meter perpendicular to your mouth.
- Take a deep breath in.
- Cover the mouthpiece with your lips to form a tight seal.
- Blow out as fully and quickly as possible.

Take the best reading of three attempts and plot on a chart of daily results.

Uses

This is a simple but effective measure of lung function, especially in asthmatic patients. Such patients should know their best peak flow reading when they are in good health.

The test should be conducted on a daily basis and the results plotted. Because asthmatic patients usually experience a 'morning dip' in their reading when they are unwell, they should measure their flow rate in the morning and evening. A dip of 20% is a warning sign of an exacerbation and the patient should visit their GP for a check-up. According to British Thoracic Society Guidelines, a peak flow of 50% of the patient's best (or predicted) reading indicates the need for admission to hospital. When assessing peak flow rates in hospital, readings should ideally be taken pre- and post-nebuliser/inhaler use. Criteria for discharge include a peak flow rate of greater than 80%.

Peak flow readings can also be used as a baseline in spirometry.

Spirometry

This is a lung function test where values are obtained of lung volume and flow rate.

There are many facets to spirometry, the basic test involves measuring the forced expired volume of air in 1 s (FEV_1) and forced vital capacity (FVC). The ratio (FEV_1/FVC) is then calculated. A normal ratio is about 4 : 5, or 80%.

Obstructive spirometry

The FEV_1 is reduced in obstructive spirometry, as is the FEV_1/FVC ratio.

Causes
- Asthma
- Bronchial carcinoma
- Chronic obstructive pulmonary disease (COPD).

Restrictive spirometry

Here, the FVC is reduced but the FEV_1/FVC ratio is normal.

Causes
- Lung fibrosis
- Kyphosis
- Pulmonary oedema
- Pleural effusion.

6

Asthma – inhaler technique

Please explain and demonstrate the use of inhalers for the treatment of asthma.

Answer follows . . .

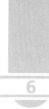

6

Asthma – inhaler technique

Answer

This is a deceptively easy station; however, marks may be lost for not stating things that may seem simple and obvious to you.

Note: Make sure you are familiar with the current British Thoracic Society guidelines for the stepwise treatment of asthma.

There are four sections to explaining this technique:

1. The need for an inhaler
2. Demonstration of the technique
3. Dosage and side-effects
4. Time to answer the patient's/family's questions and concerns.

Steps

1. Explain, in simple terms (if the patient does not already know) that asthma is a narrowing of the airways, causing difficulties in breathing. Inhalers help to ease breathing by widening the airways. The β_2 agonist (blue inhaler, 'reliever') achieve this quickly and should be used whenever symptoms occur, such as with exercise or cold weather. It may also be advisable to use the blue inhaler immediately before exercise. Steroids (brown inhaler, 'preventer') are used for prophylaxis, and should be taken every day regardless of symptoms.
Inhalers are used in preference to oral preparations

because the direct delivery to the lungs allows for a lower dosage, thus reducing possible side-effects.

2. Demonstrate the technique as follows:
    - (a) remove the cap
    - (b) shake the inhaler
    - (c) breathe out completely
    - (d) place the inhaler in your mouth, securing your lips around the mouthpiece
    - (e) begin to breathe in deeply, activating the inhaler as you do so
    - (f) complete the inhalation and hold your breath for 10 s
    - (g) breathe normally
    - (h) repeat Steps (b)–(h) for the second dose.

Ask the patient to demonstrate the technique back to you. Correct any problems before moving onto Step 3.

3. The blue inhaler (which should be carried with the patient at all times) is usually prescribed as 'two puffs when needed' – no more than eight puffs should be taken in 24 h. The brown inhaler provides a fixed daily dose, which may need increasing if symptoms are not controlled.

The patient should be made aware that blue inhalers (β_2 agonist) may cause tremor and headache. Because the brown (steroid) inhaler can lead to oral candidiasis, it is advisable to wash the mouth after each use. Higher doses of steroids can result in stunting of growth. In children, they are often prescribed for use on alternate days.

4. Time should be left for the patient (or their family) to ask questions at the end. Asthma can be a stigmatising condition, and the importance of complying with the treatment should be stressed. Similarly, the patient should not keep increasing their treatment if symptoms are not controlled – they should be advised to see their doctor for alteration of therapy. Anxious patients may need to be

reassured that systemic side-effects are very rare with inhaled steroids, and only occur at very high doses.

A note on spacers

Some patients find it difficult to follow the correct inhaler technique (particularly the very young and the very old), but adding a plastic spacer ensures that an effective dose still reaches the lungs. One end of the spacer attaches to the inhaler mouthpiece, the other end (which the patient puts in their mouth) contains a one-way valve. After activating the inhaler, the patient breathes normally for 30 seconds through the spacer; the process is then repeated for the second dose.

7

Venepuncture

Mr Manning is a known insulin dependent diabetic on the morning list for a left-sided inguinal hernic repair. Please take the relevant pre-operative blood samples.

It is better not to address the manikin used for this station, but do speak to the examiner (unless otherwise specified).

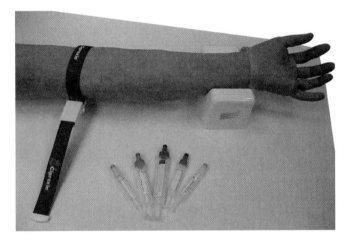

Figure 5.7

Answer follows . . .

Venepuncture

Answer

A simple case scenario will be presented and you must use your common sense as to which blood tests you would like to request for the patient. For example:
- a patient going for surgery will need a full blood count, clotting parameters, group and save serum.
- a post-operative patient or a patient on medication may need U&E (urea and electrolytes) monitoring, and
- a known diabetic would require a glucose estimation.

There are some special blood tests that you should bear in mind, e.g.:

- people of African origin may need a sickle-cell test if their status is unknown
- an older woman with a headache may need an ESR measurement
- a patient on warfarin will require an INR
- a patient known to be actively bleeding will need an urgent cross-match.

Steps

1. Tell the examiner you would introduce yourself to the patient. Explain that you would like to take a sample of blood for a blood test(s). This will mean a 'sharp scratch', but it should be over very quickly. Say you would obtain the patient's permission to carry on.
2. Before proceeding, check the patient's identity with

their hospital number (on their identity bracelet). If the manikin doesn't have a bracelet (or number elsewhere), tell the examiner you would do this check.

3. Select your equipment: a needle/Vacutainer (see below), blood-test tubes (see below), gloves, cotton-wool pad/gauze, alcohol wipes, tourniquet, adhesive dressing (Elastoplast), blood-test request forms and plastic self-seal bags. **Ensure a sharps bin is positioned nearby** (i.e. as close as possible) **before starting**.

4. Look for a good vein on the manikin, and apply the tourniquet a few centimetres above.

5. Put on your gloves and clean the site with an alcohol wipe.

6. Place the needle or introduce the Vacutainer bevel up into the vein, forewarn the patient of a sharp scratch sensation.

7. Allow the 'blood' to fill the tubes (a fair amount in each tube, there is usually a marker on the label).

8. Remove the tourniquet and **then** the needle. **Dispose of the needle into the sharps bin**.

9. Quickly place a cotton-wool or gauze pad over the wound. Advise the patient to apply pressure for some time.

10. During this time ask the patient if s/he has an allergy to adhesive dressings (Elastoplast). Label the blood tubes (details below) and place the tubes and forms in the plastic self-seal bags as provided.

11. Cover the puncture site with an adhesive dressing. Thank the patient.

12. Turn to the examiner and beam a smile!

Discussion

Types of needle available

In the UK, two basic types of venepuncture kit are available:

- **Monovac**: This is a needle to which various blood tubes

can be attached and detached via plastic grips.
- **Vacutainer**: This is a needle with a plastic hub, to which tubes can be attached and detached.

The type you will be given will depend on where your PLAB examination takes place. Although it may be a little different from what you are used to, it doesn't really matter – at the end of the day, it's just a matter of drawing blood.

Blood tubes

Again, different parts of the country use different coloured blood tubes. Instead of memorising colours, you will probably find it more useful to know which preservative the tube contains:
- FBC (full blood count): EDTA
- U&E (urea and electrolytes): serum gel

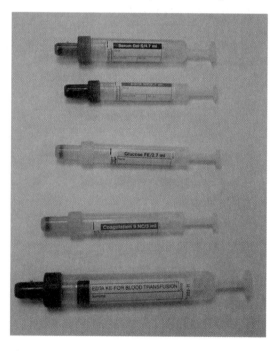

Figure 5.8

- glucose: sodium fluoride
- coagulation: contains sodium citrate.

Others
- Any other sample for chemistry/immunology tends to go in the U&E bottle.
- Any other haematology (e.g. malaria screen, sickle-cell screen) tends to go in the FBC bottle.
- Note that the ESR container will be an elongated tube/bottle.
- The Group and Save container is usually labelled as such, and tends to be the largest tube/bottle amongst the rest. It is usually a plain, preservative-free tube.

Sharps disposal
Never re-sheath any needle.
- Always place your used needle in the yellow and red plastic bin provided, called a 'sharps bin' or 'sharps safe' container.

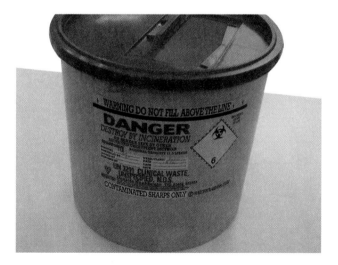

Figure 5.9

- Before starting the procedure, place the bin close to you so that you are not walking around with the needle, this is to avoid a needlestick injury. If you have already started and forgotten to place the sharps bin nearby, go ahead and ask the examiner to move it closer for you.

Blood forms

Unless it has been otherwise specified, hand-write the labels on all blood tubes and blood forms. Some hospitals provide ready-made, adhesive labels containing the patient's details. You will not fail the station for not completing the labelling process, so long as you are safe in your technique and know how to label and seal the containers. Generally, labelling requires: a patient/hospital number; the patient's name and date of birth; today's date; the ward number; your signature.

Note: The label on the Group and Save bottle should always be handwritten (national hospital policy).

8

Intravenous cannulation

Please insert an intravenous cannula into this patient who will be going to theatre.

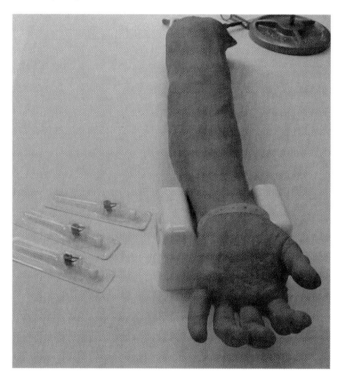

Figure 5.10

Answer follows . . .

Intravenous cannulation

Answer

A manikin will be used for this station.

An intravenous cannula (often called by the trade name 'Venflon') is a means of gaining intravenous (iv) access.

Different gauge cannulas are available, ranging in size from 14 (very wide bore) to 24 (very fine bore, but large enough for delivering antibiotics intravenously). When given a choice, and if a vein permits, opt for an 18–20-gauge cannula. A larger cannula size should be selected for resuscitation purposes, or for patients who will be undergoing surgery.

This is the usual instruction for this station, so opt for a larger size cannula and explain your reasoning (note that the much larger sizes may be more difficult to insert in the manikin, so choose the size you know you can handle).

Steps

1. Tell the examiner you would introduce yourself to the patient.
2. Explain you need to gain access to the vein so that medication or fluids or blood can be put directly in the system, which is beneficial to the patient. This means that a small plastic tube will be put in the arm, it will hurt a little bit, but it will be over very quickly. Say you would obtain the patient's permission to proceed.
3. Select your equipment: gloves, cannula, 10 ml saline

flush, a means to fix the cannula (clear adhesive dressing, e.g. Tegaderm or Vecafix), a tourniquet, gauze, alcohol wipes and a 10 ml syringe. **Place a sharps bin close to you.**
4. Check the patient's identity bracelet.
5. Keeping your equipment close by, draw up the flush, and open the gauze, adhesive and cannula packages.
6. Select a vein, tighten the tourniquet a few centimetres above, put on your gloves and clean the area with an alcohol wipe.
7. Remove the plastic cover from the cannula needle, remove the cap and keep it handy, then quickly flip the port lid to ensure it is working.
8. Take your time and place the cannula, look for the flashback. Once you have a flashback stop moving the needle and continue to advance the plastic tube until it is completely inserted.
9. When you are satisfied, remove the needle and place it in the sharps bin, replace the cap and secure the cannula. (Keep some cotton-wool or gauze handy to mop up any spillages.)
10. Remove the tourniquet.
11. Flush the cannula.
12. Tell the examiner you would thank the patient.
13. Turn to the examiner.

Discussion

Parts of the cannula

A cannula comprises a needle (i.e. an introducer) and a plastic component; on top of the latter there is a port (for iv injections), and at the back there is a connection through which fluids/blood may be introduced. The needle will be covered by a plastic sheath.

Flush

It is important to show that you have checked the 10 ml

ampoule of normal saline along with its expiry date, after all you are going to inject this intravenously. What if it was actually a 10 ml bottle of lidocaine (lignocaine) that had been placed there accidentally? The label must always be checked carefully (preferably double-checked with another member of staff), both for your own safety and that of the patient.

9

Intravenous and intramuscular injections

Please give an iv injection of metoclopramide through the cannula in this patient.

Answer follows . . .

Intravenous and intramuscular injections

Answer

Yet another deceptively simple station! However, there are many common pitfalls that must be avoided.

The case will be something simple, unless the examiner is also trying to test your knowledge of drugs. In this case the injection is to be a commonly used anti-emetic, metoclopramide. The dose is 10 mg iv. **Remember** that metoclopramide is contraindicated in children (possible dystonic reactions) and in those suffering from parkinsonism. Rule out any individual drug allergies by checking the patient's drug chart and wrist band. Assuming none of the above are applicable you may proceed.

Steps

1. Check the patient's ID, and confirm this with the patient's identity bracelet.
2. Ensure iv access is available.
3. Explain to the patient that you would like to give her a drug to help control her vomiting.
4. Ask the patient about any drug allergies. Obtain her permission to proceed.
5. Put on a pair of gloves.
6. Select a vial of metoclopramide, check the name, quantity, concentration and expiry date of the contents.
7. Double-check the above details with another member of

the medical or nursing staff.

8. Break open the glass ampoule along the dotted line at its neck. Draw up the metoclopramide into a syringe fitted with a green needle.

9. Draw up a flush of 10 ml normal saline into a 10 ml syringe.

10. Double-check the name, quantity and expiry date of the normal saline with a colleague.

11. Open the cannula port and inject the metoclopramide as a rapid bolus over a few seconds.

12. Follow by injecting the saline flush.

13. Ensure that all sharps (needles, glass ampoules and vials) have been disposed of into a **nearby sharps bin**, and contaminated cotton-wool, etc. into the appropriate Biohazard container.

14. Thank the patient and your colleague.

Discussion

Some intravenous drugs cannot be given quickly and either require injection as a slow fluid (over 2–5 minutes) or as an infusion. If you are unsure whether or not a drug can be given as a rapid bolus, check with a colleague or look in a recent copy of the BNF (*British National Formulary*).

Intramuscular injection

An im injection is very similar in principle, except that the bulk of the deltoid or gluteal muscles are used instead. A stabbing technique is assumed; remember to pinch up the muscle beforehand.

10

Measuring blood pressure

Please measure this patient's blood pressure.

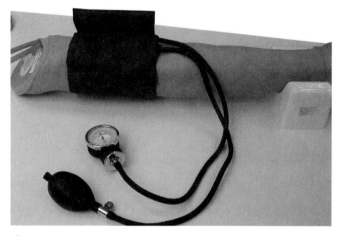

Figure 5.11

Answer follows . . .

Measuring blood pressure

Answer

On the surface, this is a seemingly simple station. However, it is surprising how easily an error can be made, especially when you are under pressure.

Note: If a manikin is used in this station the examiner can set the blood pressure (BP) reading beforehand, so don't guess the reading, try to be as accurate as possible.

Checkpoints for this station include:
- correct technique
- correct instruction
- adequate reading (another stethoscope is available for the examiner to check the reading)
- discussion (usually postural hypotension in a known diabetic patient or recommended thresholds for diagnosing hypertension – currently > 140/90 mmHg).

Steps

1. Introduce yourself to the patient.
2. Explain that you are about to measure their blood pressure. Say that a cuff will be wrapped around the arm and pressure applied, and, although it may feel a little uncomfortable, it should not hurt.
3. Once the patient understands, obtain their permission to proceed.
4. Select the cuff size (show the examiner you are doing this; see 'Discussion' below for details).

5. Attach the equipment and check that the sphygmomanometer is working.

6. Wrap the cuff around the patient's arm, with the bladder over the brachial artery.

7. The arm should be at the level of the heart (rest the arm on a nearby table, or ask for support if one is not available).

8. Palpate the radial/brachial artery while increasing the pressure, note the systolic pressure when the pulse disappears – this is the **palpatory method**.

9. Allow the cuff to deflate fully as you place the stethoscope over the brachial artery.

10. Re-inflate the cuff to 20 mmHg above the systolic reading you found by the palpatory method.

11. To then measure blood pressure by the **auscultatory method**, deflate the cuff slowly (2 mmHg per second) and listen for the point at which the sounds appear (Korotkof I) indicating systolic pressure, continue to release slowly until the sounds disappear (Korotkof V).

12. Deflate the cuff. Say you would like to rule out postural hypotension. Tell the patient that you would like to repeat the procedure with them standing. Say they must stand **slowly**, and they should hold on to the table for support if they feel giddy or light-headed (**important instruction**.)

13. Repeat the procedure.

14. Note the measurements and turn to the examiner to relay your findings.

Discussion

Size of the cuff

- There are likely to be three cuff sizes available, basically: large, medium and small. More precisely, these sizes correspond to the bladder being approximately two-thirds the diameter of the patient's upper arm.

- If a cuff is too tight (e.g. in obese people) it may result in increased pressure over the artery and a false high reading. Too loose (e.g. in thin children), and the reading may be inaccurately low.
- A larger cuff is available for measuring blood pressure in the lower limb.

When to repeat a BP measurement

- Repeat the BP measurement in the opposite arm if a dissecting thoracic/abdominal aortic aneurysm is suspected.
- Repeat the BP measurement in a lower limb if coarctation of the aorta is suspected.
- Blood pressures are repeated over time when diagnosing hypertension (on three separate occasions).
- Repeat the standing/lying/sitting blood pressure measurements to eliminate postural hypotension this is often the theme of the station.

Postural hypotension

Definition

A systolic BP drop of more than 20 mmHg indicates postural hypotension.

Symptoms

- Patient feels light-headed/dizzy/giddy when standing too quickly, or getting out of bed.
- Patient has sycopal attacks.

Causes

- Hypovolaemia: dehydration, blood loss (post-operatively)
- Drugs: nitrates, calcium-channel blockers, tricyclic antidepressants
- Autonomic neuropathy: diabetes, amyloidosis, Parkinson's disease-related, vasculitis.

Further information

Please consult The British Hypertension Society Guidelines website.

11

Rectal examination

Perform a rectal examination on an anatomical model, assuming it to be a real patient. Describe your findings to the examiner.

Answer follows . . .

11

Rectal examination

Answer

A manikin will be used for this station. In the past, the manikin has been set up to have, for example, an enlarged prostate – so make sure you do the station properly (and not just go through the motions) because you will be asked questions at the end.

Steps

1. Explain that you would introduce yourself to the patient. Ensure adequate privacy before conducting the procedure and ask for a chaperone. Say you would explain to the patient that you need to examine their back passage, that this may be uncomfortable but should not be painful, and you will stop immediately if it is too painful. Tell the examiner you would obtain patient's consent to proceed.
2. Gather your equipment – including: gloves (no need to be sterile), lubricating gel, a good light source and some tissues to wipe down the patient.
3. Ask the patient to lie in the left lateral position, to undress from the waist down and to try to relax.
4. Inspection – look for: any rash/excoriation; any polyps, prolapsed piles, perianal haematoma, carcinoma, etc; any scars or obvious fistulas; any ulcers or fissures.
5. Palpation – having applied plenty of lubricating gel, place the pulp of your right index finger on the centre of the anus, gently press inwards and backwards.
6. Note the tone of the anal sphincter. Any pain? Any masses?

7. Feel inside the rectum for any masses or ulcers, or any faeces. Go as high as you can.

8. Turn your finger around so that the pulp of your finger is facing forwards, then feel for the rectovesico or rectouterine pouch (pouch of Douglas). Are there any masses or fluid?

9. Complete the examination by conducting a bimanual examination, place your left hand over the abdomen to examine the contents of the pelvis.

10. After removing your finger, inspect it for blood, mucus and faeces.

11. Mention that you would thank the patient for their co-operation and ask them to get dressed.

Discussion

Prostate

- In a male patient you would be able to feel the prostate gland, which is normally smooth and rubbery and about 2–3 cm across.
- In the case of benign prostatic hypertrophy, although it will remain firm and smooth, the prostate will be much enlarged; there may be a preceding history of difficulty in micturition/stream.
- In the case of malignancy, the mass is likely to be hard and irregular, and the rectal mucosa may be fixed to the underlying gland.

Uterus, etc

- In a female patient it is possible to feel the uterus, and the trained person can define its shape and size.
- Bimanual palpation may help you to identify any enlarged adnexal masses.

Rectum

- The rectum is normally empty or 'boggy' filled with faeces.

- If a hard mass is palpable in the rectum, it is suspicious and needs investigation.

Faeces

The colour of the faeces and the presence of any blood or mucus is very helpful for your differential diagnosis.

Pain

- The presence of pain when initially entering the rectum indicates anal fissures, therefore the examination should be stopped immediately if it is too painful.
- Pain while palpating inside the rectum may sometimes indicate an inflamed appendix, correlate this finding with the patient's history.

12

Vaginal examination

Perform a bimanual vaginal examination on an anatomical model, assuming it to be a real patient. Describe your findings to the examiner (a speculum or smear examination is not required).

Answer follows . . .

12

Vaginal examination

Answer

This is a typical GMC PLAB Part 2 question. As always, it is important to read the question first and follow the instructions given. Remember that you only have 5 minutes to complete the station, so stick to the task you've been asked to perform as you will only be assessed on that. However, all aspects of the different tasks normally encountered in the gynaecological examination will be covered below.

As a general rule, it is very important to identify the patient in the examination room, as the last thing you want to do is perform an unnecessary examination on the wrong patient. So if the patient's name is mentioned on the task card, start by saying: 'Good morning Mrs Smith, I'm Dr Banerjee, one of the doctors working in the obstetrics and gynaecology department of this hospital'.

It is **absolutely essential** that you are accompanied by a chaperone when performing any intimate gynaecological examination, irrespective of whether you are male or female. Remember it is quite different examining an anatomical model and a real patient, so you must perform the examination with the same dignity and sensitivity you would normally employ in a real-life scenario.

Examination

- Reassure the patient before you start that the procedure

is not painful, as such, but it may be a little uncomfortable.

- Explain that you will perform a digital internal examination with one hand while keeping your other hand on the top of the lower part of her tummy. Say that it helps us to find out if there is anything wrong with her reproductive organs.
- It is vitally important to obtain the patient's verbal consent for any such procedure, and it is wise to mention the fact in the notes.
- Make sure the patient has emptied her bladder before examining her.

Bimanual vaginal examination

- Follow the instructions above.
- Introduce yourself to the patient, checking you have the right patient (see above).
- Ensure a chaperone is present and that privacy is maintained at all times.
- Ask the patient to undress from the waist down and then lie down on the couch.
- By this time, you should have your examination trolley ready. Make sure it contains: a pair of gloves in your size (need not be sterile); a tube of lubricating K-Y jelly; a chlamydial endocervical swab and a high vaginal swab if you are going to do an infection screen; a cervical brush or an Ayre's wooden spatula, a glass slide and a fixative spray if you going to perform a cervical smear (don't forget a pencil for labelling the slide, lab. request forms and plastic specimen bags); and a Cusco's bivalved speculum. (*It might be worthwhile mentioning to the examiner that, ideally, you would first examine the patient's abdomen before proceeding to the vaginal examination.*)
- Get the patient to lie in the proper examination position by asking her to bend her knees and put her heels

together and then flop her knees apart to expose the introitus (don't say 'introitus' to the patient as they unlikely to know what you mean).

- Don your gloves and then place a small amount of K-Y jelly on the tip of the index and middle fingers of your right hand. With your left thumb and index finger, part the labia and proceed to examine the patient with the middle and index fingers of your right hand while keeping your thumb extended and your little and ring fingers flexed.

- Start your discussion by commenting on your observations of the external genitalia. Mention any excoriations, growths, warts and leucoplakia, etc.

- Then, while keeping your hand on the patient's suprapubic region, comment on the position of the uterus – whether it is anteverted or retroverted. (*However, it's sometimes difficult to comment on this in an anatomical model*). Then state whether the size of the uterus is normal or bulky.

- Comment on the adnexal pathology, whether you can feel for any swelling or tenderness in the right or left fornix. Remember to move your other hand on the left and right iliac fossa while looking for the corresponding adnexal tenderness or mass.

- Finally comment on any cervical excitation and mass or nodules in the Pouch of Douglas. When looking for cervical excitation gently push the cervix to one side while looking at the patient's face for any sign that she's feeling discomfort.

- End by giving the patient a tissue to wipe herself and telling her that she can put on her clothes.

- Thank the patient.

- Explain your bimanual vaginal examination findings to the examiner. Tell him/her that in a real-life scenario you would inform the patient of your findings.

Speculum and cervical smears

If you were asked to take a speculum or a cervical smear then follow the same initial steps: ask the patient to lie in the same position and explain to her what each examination will entail. In a speculum examination we look at the neck of the womb for any cervical pathology, any cervical dilatation or product of conception in the os in a threatened/incomplete/inevitable miscarriage. For a cervical smear we use the same instrument to visualise the neck of the womb and take a smear from it using the cervical brush or the Ayre's wooden spatula; this is part of the national screening programme for cervical cancers.

You are expected to use the Cusco's bivalved speculum when performing a **speculum examination**:

- Forewarn the patient that the speculum might be cold but you will try and warm it in warm water.
- Before going ahead with the examination, make sure the speculum is in the proper position and that it is completely unscrewed to allow the blades to open completely.
- Once again, part the labia using the thumb and index finger of your left hand. Using your right hand, insert the speculum so the blades are facing down and the screw is facing upwards. Gently open the blades of the speculum, looking at the cervix at all times so that it lies between the upper and the lower blade. Once the cervix is properly centred fix the speculum by tightening the screw. (Don't forget to look at the patient's face for signs of pain/discomfort.)
- Comment on the local pathology that you see on the cervix, e.g. a polyp or erosion. Also make a note of any vaginal discharge or bleeding.

If you are asked to perform a **cervical smear** then proceed from here onwards using an Ayre's wooden spatula or cervical brush.

- Using the bi-grooved end of an Ayre's speculum (the other end is flat), rotate the spatula five times clockwise along the neck of the womb to obtain a cervical smear. Spread the smear onto a glass slide and fix it by spraying with the fixative (don't forget to label the slide fully). If the woman is menopausal, a cervical brush is used in exactly the same way. (Recently, we have started using a different technique called 'liquid-based cytology' to process the slides and obtain a more accurate smear result. It is presently being conducted as a pilot study in a few centres all over the country and has been shown to greatly reduce false-positive results.)
- Unscrew the speculum and gently remove it from the vagina, making sure that no skin or tissue gets caught between the blades. Be particularly careful not to catch the cervix between the blades.
- Give a tissue to the patient to wipe herself and ask her to get dressed.
- Tell the patient that it normally takes about 14 days to get the results back, and she will either receive a letter from the hospital or her GP will inform her of the results.
- End by thanking the patient for her kind co-operation.

Data interpretation and emergency management

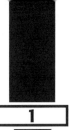

1

How to interpret a chest X-ray

Most chest X-rays are taken as a PA (posteroanterior) projection: the patient stands erect with their chest and sternum nearest to the film, their shoulders are brought forwards so the scapulas can be projected off the chest. The X-ray tube is positioned behind the patient and there is little in the way of geometric magnification of the heart size on the resulting film. Not all patients, however, are able to be adequately radiographed in this position. An X-ray of a patient supine or sitting up in bed results in an AP (anteroposterior) film, in which there is some magnification of the heart and mediastinum and the scapulas overlie the upper zones. It is important to check the X-ray is correctly labelled with the patient's name and date of the examination. Conventionally, this information appears at the top right-hand side on a PA film. It is also important to check the side markers since, although rather rare, dextrocardia or situs inversus is occasionally encountered.

A systematic approach is needed to assess the vast amount of information contained on a conventional X-ray. If the patient is well positioned with respect to the film, the medial ends of the clavicles will be seen to be equidistant from the vertebral spinous processes. If the patient is rotated to one side then the right heart border can be obscured, or the mediastinum may appear unduly widened.

A systematic approach to assessing an X-ray

The following points should be considered:
• heart size, contour and silhouette

- both hemidiaphragms
- mediastinal structures, including the aorta and trachea
- hilar regions
- lungs, pulmonary vessels, lung edge
- areas of increased opacity, nodules and masses, linear shadows
- loss of the silhouette sign of the heart mediastinum and hemidiaphragms
- bony structures: ribs, vertebrae and shoulder girdle

Silhouette sign

The appearances of the heart, mediastinum and lungs mainly depend on the differences in trans-radiance of the air-containing lung adjacent to the soft tissues of heart, the

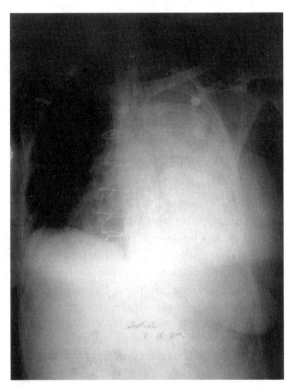

Figure 6.1

mediastinum and the pulmonary vessels. The aerated lung adjacent to the heart along the right heart border and left heart border enables the cardiac contour to be clearly seen.

The left heart border in Fig. 6.1 is not seen because the whole of the left lung is no longer aerated. In this patient, who has recently undergone aortic valve replacement, this is due to aspirated fluid and secretions filling the alveoli. Note the presence of metallic sternal sutures and the wire struts of the aortic replacement.

Case scenario – 1

A 25-year-old tall, thin, asthmatic man presents to you with a sudden episode of shortness of breath. You treat him with nebulisers and oxygen. What abnormality (if any) does his chest X-ray show?

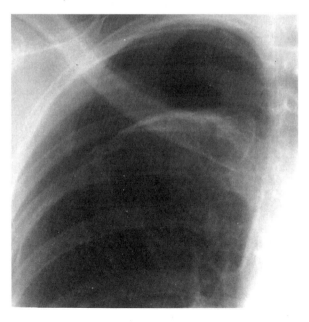

Figure 6.2

Discussion

In this chest X-ray there is an apical pneumothorax and the lung edge can be seen 3–4 cm away from the ribs at the apex. Pulmonary vessels are not seen in this area.

The heart

The transverse diameter of the heart is normally less than 50% of the maximum transverse diameter of the chest, taken from the inner margins of the ribs laterally at their widest point. The heart appears larger on supine or AP films. Superiorly, the right heart border is made up of the superior vena cava and the right atrium, which are separated by the pericardium and pleura from the right middle lobe. The left heart border is seen in its lower portion because of the normal aerated lung of the lingular lobe. Superiorly, the left heart border is made up of the main pulmonary outflow tract and the aortic knuckle. These are clearly seen because there is an aerated lung in the left upper lobe.

Mediastinum and hila

The trachea is seen as an air-filled structure lying centrally. However, it is often displaced slightly to the right by the aorta, particularly in older patients. A good quality X-ray should allow the right and left main bronchi to be visible, and the normal carinal angle between the right and left main bronchi should be less than 90°.

The hila are made up of the pulmonary arteries and pulmonary veins and the bronchi at the root of the lung. The right hemidiaphragm is usually slightly higher than the left.

Lungs

The only clearly visible structures within the lungs are the pulmonary arteries and veins; normally, these are seen to extend as far as the outer third of the lung parenchyma. The lower zone vessels are usually slightly more prominent than the upper zone vessels on the PA film, as a result of the normal differential blood flow. The lung edge cannot be seen in the normal patient since it is in contact with the chest wall and can only be seen in the presence of a pneumothorax. The fissures separating the left upper and lower lobes and the right upper, middle and lower lobes are not usually visible, with the exception of the horizontal fissure on the right that extends from the right hilum to the chest wall and marks the upper border of the right middle lobe.

Bones and soft tissues

Bony structures, including the ribs, clavicles and (usually) the shoulder girdle, are visible on the PA film and attention should be paid to these. Overlying soft tissue abnormalities may occasionally cause confusion. In females, the breasts may produce significant soft tissue shadowing over the lower zones and nipple shadows may occasionally be mistaken for a pulmonary lesion.

Abnormalities that should be looked for on a chest X-ray

- An increase in heart size
- Loss of the normal silhouette of the cardiac contour (see Fig. 6.1) or diaphragm due to the absence of aerated lung adjacent to these structures
- Areas of increased density
- Rounded lesions and linear shadows.

Case senario – 2

A 40-year-old woman on long-term steroids for rheumatoid arthritis is referred to you from her GP. She has a 2-week history of cough and sputum. She has become progressively unwell, and has developed shortness of breath (sats 80% on air) and a tight wheezy chest with decreased breath sounds. She is also pyrexial 38 °C. What is your diagnosis from her chest X-ray?

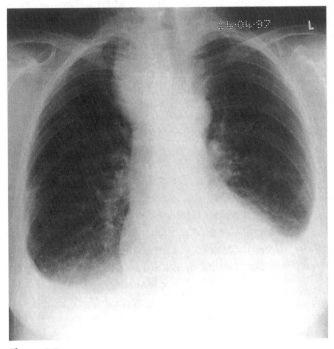

Figure 6.3

Discussion

Consolidation

'Consolidation' is the term used to describe a section of lung, an entire lobe or, occasionally, a whole lung where the alveoli are no longer aerated. In this situation they may be filled with fluid, pus, tumour cells or even blood.

It is impossible on a chest X-ray to determine the nature of the material that has replaced the air. One feature of a consolidated lung is that the major airways into the affected area still contain air, an appearance termed an 'air bronchogram'. Small quantities of fluid in the pleural space are seen as blunting of the costophrenic angles (see the X-ray of this man's chest), but more extensive fluid will produce an opacity of the lower zones or even complete opacification of the hemithorax. Radiologically, it is not possible to differentiate between pleural transudates, exudates, blood or chyle within the pleural space.

Case scenario – 3

An 86-year-old Asian woman presents to you with significant weight loss, night sweats and haemoptysis. What conclusion would you draw from her chest X-ray?

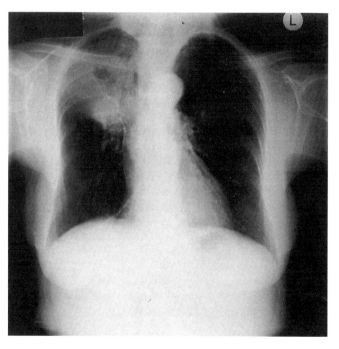

Figure 6.4

Discussion

Masses and nodules

When assessing rounded lesions, comment on:

- the size of the lesion
- the contour (is it well defined or are the edges indistinct or spiculated?)
- the number of lesions (single or multiple?)
- the density (soft tissue fluids, or is calcification present?)

This woman's X-ray shows a well-defined mass lesion in the right upper zone abutting the right side of the superior mediastinum, the right hilar vessels are not seen through the mass. A small pocket of air is seen within the mass, indicating the mass is cavitating. Multiple, small (1–2 mm), rounded opacities scattered throughout both lungs are often described as 'miliary opacities'.

2

How to interpret an electrocardiogram

The electrocardiogram should be interpreted in a stepwise fashion. Make sure the calibration signal is on the tracing and that it is exactly 1 cm (which equals 1 mV). The tracing should be repeated if the calibration signal is distorted, this is because it can cause artefacts that may be misinterpreted as a pathological change.

Make sure you check the name and, if possible, the age of the patient.

Modern machines in casualty departments often incorporate a computer program that analyses the tracings. The programs occasionally make mistakes, but it is worthwhile reading the computer interpretation and checking it with your own report.

Main axis

Normally, we only look at the main deflection of the QRS complex. However, it is also important to look at the axis of the P- and T-waves, which should, with minor variations, be about the same as the QRS complexes.

The main axis can easily be estimated by looking at leads I, II and III:
- If you find positive (upward) deflections of the QRS complexes in leads I and II, the axis is normal.
- If only lead I has a major positive deflection, the condition is called 'left anterior hemi-block' or 'left axis deviation'.

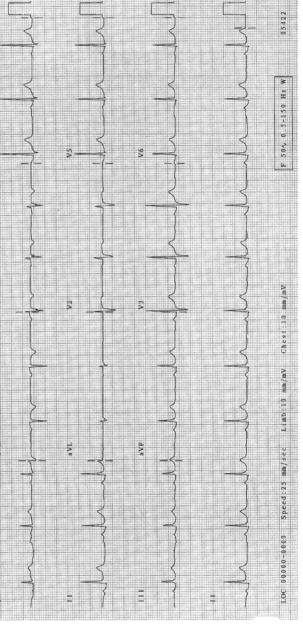

Figure 6.5 ECG of normal sinus rhythm.

- If the only positive deflection is in lead II and/or III, there is right axis deviation.

Rhythm and rate

British electrocardiograms are recorded at a speed of 25 mm/s. A simple way to assess the heart rate is to divide 300 by the number of large squares (5-mm squares) between two QRS complexes. Rates under 60 and above 100 are regarded as abnormal (i.e. the distance between two QRS complexes should not be less than three large squares and not more than five large squares).

The next thing is to check is if the heart rhythm is regular. The commonest abnormality is atrial fibrillation. If there are any doubts about the regularity of the rhythm use a paper strip: mark three complexes, then slide the paper slip along the tracing and compare the distance between other QRS complexes.

Occasionally, it is difficult to diagnose atrial fibrillation because minor changes of the baseline are visible, suggestive of P-waves. P-waves are normally best seen in leads II and V1; if they change their form from beat to beat you are dealing with either an atrial tachycardia or with atrial fibrillation. The distinction between the two states is basically a question of definition and two conditions can show up in the same tracing.

It is important not to miss bradycardia (under 60 beats/min) or tachycardia (over 100 beats/min).

If you encounter bradycardia you are dealing either with sinus bradycardia or with a conduction defect in the atrioventricular (AV) node (e.g. third-degree heart block). Note that third-degree heart block often coincides with slow atrial fibrillation and therefore the QRS sequence is irregular.

If you encounter tachycardia it is important to distinguish

between broad- and narrow-complex tachycardia.
Broad-complex tachycardia is usually due to ventricular
tachycardia, which is a medical emergency.

P-wave and P-R interval

After you have established the rate and rhythm, assess the
P-wave and P-R interval.

P-waves

These should be no higher than 2.5 mm and no wider than
3 mm. If you find wider P-waves you are probably dealing
with a so-called 'P-mitrale', which indicates left atrial
enlargement due to mitral valve disease. In these
circumstances you will commonly find a biphasic P-wave
in V1 with a prominent negative (downwards) component.

A P-wave higher than 2.5 mm is called a 'pulmonary
P-wave' or 'P-pulmonale'. It indicates right heart disease
with pulmonary hypertension.

A 'saw-tooth' pattern in lead V1 is the hallmark of atrial
flutter.

P-R interval

Next, check the P-R interval.
- P-R interval prolongation of more than one large square
  is called 'AV block, first degree'.
- If you see a P-R interval that progressively gets longer
  followed by an isolated P-wave you are dealing with a
  Wenckebach block or heart block type 2, Mobitz type 1.
- If you find a P-wave that is only followed every second,
  third or fourth time by a QRS complex you are dealing
  with a heart block type 2, Mobitz type 2.

Wenckebach block is normally regarded as a benign
condition. Mobitz type 2 often blocks progress to AV block
type 3. In AV block type 3 the P-R interval varies and the

patient is profoundly bradycardic (often under 45 beats/min). The P-waves show no relationship to the QRS complexes.

Remember that slow atrial fibrillation is not uncommon and that you will find an irregular extreme bradycardia in such patients.

In third-degree heart block you also occasionally see marked T-wave inversions. If you find very short P-R intervals (less than three small squares) you have to consider a pre-excitation syndrome (accessory-bundle conduction with intermittent narrow-complex tachycardia).

QRS complexes

Leads I, V1 and V6 are the most important for interpreting the QRS complex for bundle-branch blocks. If you find a widened QRS complex ('sugar cane') in lead I with S-T segment depression you are dealing with a left bundle-branch block (often an 'M'-shaped QRS complex in V6).

In right bundle-branch block you will find an RSR pattern in lead V1. If the QRS complex is broader than three small squares we talk about 'complete bundle-branch blocks'. If it is less than three small squares we talk about 'incomplete bundle-branch blocks'.

Very tall R-waves are found in left ventricular hypertrophy (sum of the S-wave in V1 and the R-wave in V5 or V6 > 35 mm). If you find a high R-wave in V1 (more than 6 mm) with a deep S-wave in V6 (more than 6 mm) these are signs of right ventricular hypertrophy. An R-wave taller than 1.2 cm in AVL also suggests left ventricular hypertrophy.

Remember you can also get tall R-waves in V1 in the rare isolated posterior myocardial infarction ('true posterior infarction').

Very-small-amplitude QRS complexes are found in patients with pericardial effusion, emphysema, obesity and hypothyroidism.

S-T segment

S-T segment changes are the most important finding in the electrocardiogram. The S-T segment can either be displaced upwards or downwards. Upwards displacement is found in patients with pericarditis, acute myocardial infarction and with an unusual form of angina called 'Prinzmetal angina' (coronary artery spasms). Persistent S-T segment elevations (longer than 6 months) are suggestive of a ventricular cardiac aneurysm or a hypokinetic area.

S-T segment depression is found in myocardial ischaemia, as a digoxin side-effect or in the so-called ventricular 'strain pattern' found with right or left ventricular hypertrophy. The S-T segments are also inverted in bundle-branch blocks. **Remember** you cannot diagnose myocardial ischaemia in left bundle-branch block.

T-waves

Tall, pointed, positive T-waves are found in patients with hyperkalaemia, hyperacute myocardial infarction, occasionally in pericarditis and in young healthy people.

Negative T-waves can be a sign of a sub-endocardial myocardial infarction. They are found in the resolution phase of a myocardial infarction, and in ischaemic heart disease without evidence of myocardial death.

Little positive waves after the T-waves can occur (U-waves) in patients with in hypokalaemia, and occasionally you also find them in healthy people.

Abnormalities

- Q-waves.
- Poor R-wave progression in chest leads V1-V4 are a sign of previous anterior myocardial infarction.
- An S-wave in lead I, Q-wave in lead III and inverted T-wave in lead III suggest pulmonary embolism, but be careful with the diagnosis if the patient is not tachycardic.
- Delta waves in the QRS complex are found in patients with a pre-excitation syndrome.

Always remember that electrocardiographic abnormalities can occur in normal people without organic heart disease. Organic heart disease, however, may be present despite a normal electrocardiogram.

How to interpret blood results (1)

Mrs White, a 75-year-old woman, has presented to her GP complaining of increasing tiredness over the last 6 months. On examination she is pale and has 6 cm of splenomegaly. Her investigations are as follows:

Table 6.1 Results of investigations

Test	Value	Test	Value
Hb	7.2 g/dL	Urea	8.5 mmol/L
MCV	85 fL	Creatinine	100 mmol/L
WCC	2.5×10^9/L	AST	25 U/L
Platelets	45×10^9/L	ALT	23 U/L
Blood film	Teardrop-shaped red cells and occasional nucleated red cells	Urate	530 mmol/L
		ALP	98 U/L
		LDH	900 U/L
Sodium	136 mmol/L	CXR	Normal
Potassium	4.0 mmol/L	ECG	Normal sinus rhythm

What might be going on here and what further investigations might you want to do?

Answer follows . . .

How to interpret blood results (1)

Answer

Key points

The haematology results reveal a pancytopenia. Splenomegaly suggests the possibility of haematopoiesis in the spleen, rather than the bone marrow. (Start thinking of the causes of bone marrow infiltration/bone marrow hypoplasia.)

The raised serum urate and LDH levels reflect increased cell turnover. This is also evident on the blood film, which shows a leucoerythroblastic picture, with 'teardrop' poikilocytes (a classical finding in myelofibrosis).

This woman most probably has myelofibrosis; a bone marrow aspirate, giving a 'dry tap', may help to clinch the diagnosis. Myelofibrosis is characterised by progressive fibrosis of the bone marrow with the development of haematopoiesis in the liver and spleen; fibrosis is a secondary phenomenon due to megakaryocytic hyperplasia. It is a disease typically of older people and presents with an insidious onset with symptoms of anaemia, sweating, weight loss and anorexia. Gout is common due to a high cell turnover.

Treatment is largely palliative and aimed at reducing symptoms.

4

How to interpret blood results (2)

A 35-year-old woman, Miss Sharma, presented to her GP complaining of shortness of breath and tiredness, and she is pale. Her physician notes that she is anaemic. She has no history of haematemesis or malaena, but her past medical history includes rheumatoid arthritis. An abdominal examination is normal. Further investigations reveal the following results:

Table 6.2 Results of investigations

Test	Value	Test	Value
Hb	6.5 g/dL	Serum iron	12 µmol/L (normal range 14–29)
MCV	86 fL	TIBC	40 µmol/L (normal range 45–72)
MCH	28 pg	Ferritin	250 µg/L (normal range 15–200)
MCHC	33 g/dL	CXR	Normal
WCC	8.5 × 10⁹/L with a normal differential	ECG	Nil acute
Platelets	505 × 10⁹/L		

What is the most likely cause of her anaemia and what are the possible differential diagnoses for her anaemia?

Answer follows . . .

4

How to interpret blood results (2)

Answer

Key points

This patient, with only a history of rheumatoid arthritis and symptoms of anaemia, is most likely to have an anaemia of chronic disease (this occurs in patients with chronic inflammatory and malignant disease). The characteristic features are all present:

- a normochromic, normocytic anaemia
- reduced serum iron and TIBC
- raised serum ferritin (an inflammatory marker).

The differential diagnoses could include:

- **iron deficiency anaemia**, which is common in young females, especially those with a history of menorrhagia. It is important to rule this out here as GI bleeding secondary to NSAID treatment for rheumatoid arthritis should always be considered. However, some characteristic features of IDA include a microcytic hypochromic anaemia with a typically raised TIBC, signs that are absent in this patient.
- **thalassaemia trait** usually presents at an earlier age with a typically microcytic hypochromic anaemia, so the MCV is likely to be much lower. There may be splenomegaly. The diagnosis is more readily confirmed by haemoglobin electrophoresis showing a raised Hb A_2 level.

5

Emergency management of asthma

A 17-year-old young man has presented to you in A&E with progressive shortness of breath, occurring over the past few hours. He has a history of asthma and no known drug allergies. He has used his blue inhaler several times (lost count), but to no avail. There is a history of previous admissions to hospital but not to ITU. He is on beclomethasone 800 μg and salbutamol inhaler prn. He is unable to speak to you in sentences, his pulse rate is 120/min regular, his respiratory rate is 30 per minute. His peak flow on arrival is only 50 L/min (best = 450 L/min). Please assess him and state your emergency management.

Answer follows . . .

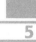

Emergency management of asthma

Answer

Steps

1. Asthma can kill, so it is important to act quickly.
   - First assess the severity of the patient's asthma.
   - Establish the vital signs immediately, regular assessment is required:
   - **mild** asthma is suggested by normal speech, a pulse rate less than 110 bpm, a respiratory rate of less than 25/min and a peak flow of greater than 50% predicted or best.
   - **severe** asthma is suggested by the patient being too wheezy or breathless to complete sentences, a pulse rate of more than 110 bpm, a respiratory rate of more than 25/min and peak flow of less than 50% of predicted normal or best.
   - **life threatening** asthma is suggested by a peak flow of less than 33% of the predicted normal or best, a silent chest, bradycardia, cyanosis, exhaustion, confusion or coma.
   - The patient mentioned in the question appears to fall into the category of severe asthma.
2. Ascertain if the patient has used any nebulisers before arriving at hospital.
   - Put the patient on a combination of oxygen and nebulisers, preferably salbutamol (5 mg stat) and Atrovent (ipratropium bromide, 500 µg stat).

3. Conduct an examination focusing on the respiratory system. It is worth ruling out a possible pneumothorax clinically.

4. Establish iv access. Administer 200 mg hydrocortisone stat.

5. It is important at this stage to attempt to gain further information, either from his relatives or the patient himself, and to re-assess the situation:

- Is the patient pyrexial, has he had a cough? If so would antibiotics be useful?
- Is there any history of trauma? (In which case a pneumothorax may be a strong possibility.)
- Rule out any history of chest pain. Request an ECG.
- Try to establish the trigger for the attack.
- Chase his old patient records to confirm no previous ITU attendances and to compare previous chest X- ray reports/ECG readings.
- Re-assess the peak flow post-nebuliser (keeping in mind the patient's best peak flow).
- Watch the oxygen saturations, if they drop below 93% on air you may consider an arterial blood gas measurement.
- It is probably wise to request a portable chest X-ray at this stage.

6. If your patient does not respond, the next line of management could include a salbutamol infusion. If the patient was already taking theophyllines then an aminophylline infusion may be appropriate. Some hospitals use continual salbutamol nebulisers. (All of the above are reasonable lines of management; it is important to know which particular method is in vogue at the time of presentation.)

7. If your patient is still not responding despite all of the above, you will need senior assistance. Do not hesitate to alert your senior doctor on duty. It may be wise to also alert ITU.

Discussion

Acute asthma is a common presentation and needs continual and rapid assessment until the patient is stable.

Management is usually straightforward – with nebulisers and oxygen – and most patients will respond. However, it is important to keep the following points in mind.

Pneumothorax

If a patient is not responding despite aggressive management, it is vital and standard practise to rule out a pneumothorax. Review the chest X-ray carefully.

Steroids

Intravenous hydrocortisone will take a few hours to act. If the patient is well, oral prednisolone may be used. Discharge the patient with a week's course of prednisolone 30 mg once-daily; advise the patient that this is not the start of long-term steroid therapy.

Salbutamol

Side-effects of salbutamol worth remembering include hypokalaemia, tremors and tachycardia, so it is necessary to keep a check on how many nebulisers the patient is receiving.

Aminophylline

Side-effects of aminophylline worth remembering include vomiting and arrhythmias. Aminophylline has a narrow therapeutic index and should be used with caution.

Infusions

The use of salbutamol or aminophylline infusion come in and out of fashion. Be familiar with updated BTS guidelines.

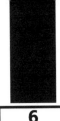

6

Emergency management of myocardial infarction

Please imagine you are an SHO working in A&E, you are on call overnight and alone, middle grade cover is available, but your staff grade is currently very busy and is unable to discuss anything with you for at least 30 minutes.

A staff nurse comes to you and shows you the following ECG (see below). The ECG belongs to a 51-year-old man, Mr Samson, who has come to the A&E department a little short of breath and complaining of chest pain. What is your diagnosis and initial management?

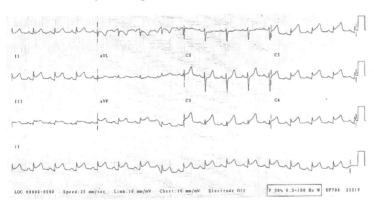

Figure 6.6

Answer follows . . .

6

Emergency management of myocardial infarction

Answer

Key points
Diagnosis and initial management

- Confirm the patient's name and the date on the ECG and then proceed to analyse it: the ECG shows an acute MI.
- Take the patient on a trolley to the resuscitation area of A&E and put him on high-flow oxygen. Monitor the patient's observations and keep him on a cardiac monitor.
- Ask the patient if he has any drug allergies in general – to aspirin in particular (e.g. gastric ulcer). If he has no problem with aspirin give him 300 mg aspirin orally.
- Give him 0.5 µg of GTN sublingually.
- Ask the staff nurse to begin cannulating the patient and to take blood samples for FBC, U&E, cardiac enzymes, lipids and glucose estimations.
- While this is happening, quickly take a **history** from the patient – asking him questions about his chest pain: type of pain, site of pain, onset of pain, duration, any relieving or aggravating factors, severity of pain on a scale of 1–10 (with 10 being the worst) and any associated features such as vomiting.
- As this is a relatively young patient, ask if there is a **family history** of cardiac problems.
- Ask the patient about his **past medical history**.
- Quickly **examine** his heart and lungs.

- Once intravenous access has been established, give the patient 2.5–5 mg diamorphine by slow iv infusion titrated to his build and level of pain, along with an iv anti-emetic, e.g. metoclopramide 10 mg iv stat.

Thrombolysis

Now that you have confirmed an MI, you need to specifically rule out **contraindications** to thrombolysis for this patient. Although you have already elicited his past medical history, specifically ask him about any:

- recent CVA
- recent trauma
- recent surgery
- recent thrombolysis (within the past 2 years)
- known allergy to thrombolytic agents
- history of high blood pressure – how high? (compare the present reading)
- history of ulcer (peptic/gastric/malaena)
- history of bleeding diathesis/clotting disorders
- severe liver disease

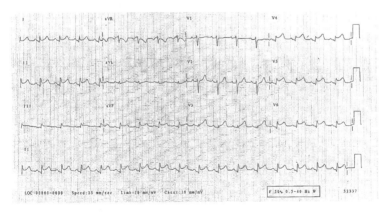

Figure 6.7

If there are no contraindications, initiate thrombolysis. Remember to make a careful note of the time and use a thrombolysing agent according to hospital policy.

Other measures

As thrombolysis proceeds, ask for a chest X-ray, notify the medical SHO on call and contact CCU with regards to bed availability. Also leave a message for your senior grade doctor so that he or she may attend if they should wish to do so.

Discussion

Question: What are the indications for thrombolysis?

Answer: Cardiac chest pain occurring within 12 hours of its onset; ST elevation > 2 mm (V1-V6) or > 1 mm (limb leads) or new Left Bundle Branch block; presence of prominent R waves and ST depression in V1-V3; presentation 12–24 hours after the onset of chest pain, still in pain with ECG evidence of evolving infarct.

Question: Name a thrombolytic agent you may use, and give its dose and route of administration.

Answer: Streptokinase 1.5 MU in 100 ml 0.9 % normal saline, iv, over 1 hour. Note that thrombolytic agents are described as 'clot busters' in lay terms.

Question: At what level of hypertension would you worry about initiating thrombolysis?

Answer: Systolic pressure > 200 mmHg; diastolic > 120 mmHg.

Question: What things would you do when you came back to review the patient?

Answer: Check the patient's observations, blood pressure, pulse rate, sats. Make sure high-flow oxygen was not compromising the patient (e.g. COPD). Complete the patient's history and examine him in more detail. Review his chest X-ray and any blood results; repeat ECG.

7

Emergency management of left ventricular failure

You are the SHO in A&E working on nights. A patient is brought in by ambulance and the crew have managed to obtain a very brief history. The patient is unable to speak in sentences.

This 88-year-old woman has become progressively short of breath over the past few days. Tonight, she went to bed feeling very tired and with some chest 'tightness', but no chest pain, only to find that she was unable to sleep. She became more and more breathless until she felt she couldn't go on any longer. Her neighbour, who had gone round to check on her, found her like this and called for an ambulance.

She is known to have heart failure, and is on 'water tablets', unfortunately no drug names are available. Initially her oxygen saturation was 85%, but with high-flow oxygen en route this improved to 90%.

How would you arrive at a diagnosis for this patient and what would be your immediate management plans.

Answer follows . . .

7

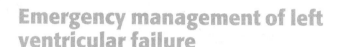

Emergency management of left ventricular failure

Answer

Key points

A good history is vital

The ambulance crew has done their best, but you need more information. Ideally, you would like to see the patient's past notes, which can be requested but may not be immediately available. Alternatively, any relatives or neighbours present at scene may be able to offer some information. You should assume that acute left ventricular failure (LVF) is the likely diagnosis.

Questions to ask the patient

- Does this patient have any other underlying medical conditions, e.g. COPD, IHD?
- Has she had a cough recently, so that LVF has been precipitated secondary to an underlying pneumonia?
- Has she had any chest pain? (Need to ask her again to rule out a possible infarct or pulmonary embolism.)
- What medications is this patient taking? Does she have any drug allergies?
- Are there any old ECG tracings? (These are useful for comparison with the present ECG in the case of ischaemic or left bundle-branch block changes.)
- Did she experience any palpitations? (LVF may be precipitated by arrhythmias such as atrial fibrillation.)

A good examination is all you have to go on!

All the above information will be available – at some point!
So it really is up to your examination skills to determine
what the problem is and what to do about it.

Observations presented to you are your key as to how ill is
the patient. You should specifically assess their **Airway –
Breathing – Circulation** (ABC):

- **Pulse:** She may be in atrial fibrillation (AF) – treat the
  underlying condition first, but remember that early
  control of the pulse rate will improve cardiac output.
- **Blood pressure:** She may well be hypertensive. A low BP
  indicates cardiogenic shock – you will need senior help.
- **Respiratory rate:** 30 and above indicates your patient is
  struggling.
- **Saturations:** Anything below 93% (or known COPD)
  would warrant arterial blood gas measurements.
- **Basal metabolism (BM):** This can be raised due to
  acidosis, treat the underlying cause if the patient is not a
  known diabetic.
- **Temperature:** Pyrexia can help you decide whether or
  not antibiotic treatment is required.

Further points

- LVF is usually a simple diagnosis clinically. The patient
  presents as being 'cool and clammy'. Any patient who is
  short of breath prefers to sit upright to open up their
  airways, but this is particularly so for a patient with
  orthopnoea due to LVF. Is the patient using accessory
  muscles of respiration?
- If the patient also has right heart failure, they will present
  with signs of fluid overload, so look for a raised JVP and
  bipedal pitting oedema.
- On palpation, rule out an underlying deep-vein
  thrombosis (DVT) in the calves and a possible
  abdominal aortic aneurysm or rigid abdomen.
- Percussion can be used to rule out any pleural effusion

or a pneumothorax.
- On auscultation, more than likely you will find coarse crepitations bi-basally. Auscultate for heart sounds – if a patient has a systolic murmur of aortic stenosis you should take care not to lower the blood pressure too quickly.

Investigations
- Arterial blood gases
- Chest X-ray
- ECG
- FBC – anaemia and infection may precipitate LVF
- U&E – the patient may also have renal disease.

Immediate management
- Sit the patient upright.
- Give high-flow oxygen.
- Gain intravenous access.
- Catheterise your patient and maintain a fluid balance.
- Use iv furosemide (frusemide) – start with 80 mg immediately, then titrate as required.
- If required, give 5 mg diamorphine iv (titrate to the patient's build and blood pressure).
- Give metoclopramide iv (anti-emetic).
- Use a salbutamol nebuliser to help to open the airways.

In real life, you will have done many of these things when assessing the patient and obtaining a good history and examination.

If upon review your patient is still struggling you may consider a nitrate infusion, but this is dependent on the patient's BP.

As you are an SHO in A&E you should discuss the case with the medical team at this stage to arrange her admission and further management.

Discussion

A lot is usually going on all at once. It is rare to come across a patient with only LVF – it is usually a combination of underlying conditions that precipitate LVF. However, for the purposes of a 5-minute OSCE it is important to be crystal clear in the basic management of a patient with LVF.

Possible questions

Question: What would you do if the patient's blood pressure did not stabilise?

Answer: In cases of low blood pressure with fluid overload the patient is in cardiogenic shock and will need a central line and possibly inotropes; this may be a case for CCU or ITU. I would call for senior assistance.

Question: What further modes of management do you know of?

Answer: Further management can include the patient requiring ventilation such as CPAP (continuous positive airways pressure), this may be a case for ITU. If LVF has been caused by an acute myocardial infarction, the patient may be a candidate for urgent thrombolysis.

Question: You cannot gain iv access, why not use oral furosemide (frusemide)?

Answer: Oral furosemide is useless in the acute situation. It is the venodilatory action of furosemide that provides instant relief rather than its diuretic action. If I really couldn't gain iv access, I would call for senior help as the patient may need a central line. Buccal or topical GTN (glyceryl trinitrate) could be used as a temporary measure in the meantime.

Question: Why do you need to catheterise in the case of SOB?

Answer: Catheterisation is often overlooked. However, it is actually a very important part of management, as otherwise a patient may be inadvertently pushed into acute renal failure. Also the patient will be very tired and unlikely to be able to cope with the diuresis without 'accidents'.

Question: What are the features to look for on a CXR of a patient with pulmonary oedema?

Answer: Cardiac enlargement; prominence of the upper lobe vessels ('upper lobe diversion'); Kerley B lines – at the bases of, or perpendicular to, the pleura; bilateral fluffy shadows in the lung fields; bilateral perihilar shadowing, often called 'bat's wing' appearance; pleural effusions or fluid in the horizontal fissure.

8

Emergency management of a pneumothorax

A 35-year-old man is admitted to Casualty with a sudden onset of shortness of breath. On examination, he is breathless at rest and centrally cyanosed with a systolic blood pressure of 100 mmHg. Examination of the chest reveals decreased expansion on the left side with absent breath sounds and hyperresonance to percussion. The trachea and apex beat are shifted towards the left.

What diagnosis should be suspected from the clinical findings?
What emergency procedure should be performed?
Discuss this man's chest X-ray.

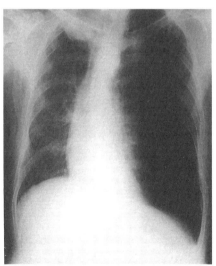

Figure 6.8

Answer follows . . .

Emergency management of a pneumothorax

Answer

- The clinical findings suggest a tension pneumothorax.
- A large-gauge needle should be inserted into the left side of his chest to release the air under tension (before requesting a chest X-ray). The needle should be placed in the second intercostal space, in the mid-clavicular line.
- The chest X-ray of this man reveals a tension pneumothorax with absent vascular markings in the periphery of the left lung, a clear lung edge can be seen and the mediastinum is shifted towards the right.

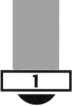

1

Morphine

Mr Cunningham is a 72-year-old man with small-cell lung cancer. He is currently taking the maximal doses of paracetamol and codeine, but he is still complaining of pain. You decide to start him on morphine. Please talk to and advise Mr Cunningham regarding morphine as an analgesic.

Answer follows . . .

Morphine

Answer

Morphine is generally used to relieve severe visceral pain, but regular use can result in tolerance or dependence (be cautious with the use of morphine in patients with sickle-cell disease).

Because morphine can give a feeling of detachment and elation, it is commonly used for pain in palliative care.

Key points

Morphine preparations

Oral

For example, Oramorph, Sevredol

- Modified-release oral preparations, e.g. MST Continus, Zomorph, MXL

Other preparations

- **Subcutaneous injections:** for acute pain (not in oedematous patients), premedication, post-operative pain (PCA, patient-controlled analgesia), chronic pain in terminal or palliative care
- **Intramuscular injections:** indications as for subcutaneous injections
- **Intravenous injections:** for acute MI by slow iv injection (2 mg/min), acute pulmonary oedema by slow iv, PCA is often given intravenously
- **Suppositories:** per rectum, can be used regularly; usually in palliative care.

Dosage

For patients in acute or chronic pain, titrate the dose against response and adverse effects. Start with 5 or 10 mg every 4 h and increase the dose as necessary. **Be aware** that morphine can accumulate in patients with renal failure.

In chronic pain, if a patient is adequately treated on oral short-acting morphine you may then convert to a once- or twice-daily regimen of a modified-release preparation. The total daily dose should be kept constant when making the change, e.g. 10 mg Oramorph every 4 h = 60 mg/day. This converts to 30 mg MST Continus twice a day, or 60 mg MXL once a day.

Side-effects

M – Miosis: therefore avoid in cases of head injury/raised intracranial pressure

O – Other: e.g. constipation, vomiting, biliary spasm, difficulty with micturition

R – Respiratory depression: therefore be cautious about opioid-induced respiratory depression

P – Palpitations: risk of exacerbating paralytic ileus (e.g. post-operatively)

H – Hypotension (and postural hypotension): hallucinations, headache.

Morphine needs to be used with an anti-emetic (e.g. cyclizine or metoclopramide) to avoid the side-effect of excessive vomiting.

Remember that naloxone is the specific antidote for morphine poisoning.

Minocycline

A young woman, who is taking minocycline to treat her acne, has read an article in a magazine about the drug's side-effects. She has come to you for advice and counselling. Please discuss the drug and your advice to this patient.

Answer follows . . .

2

Minocycline

Answer

Key points

Minocycline, a tetracycline, has predominantly been used to control severe acne, but, as with all tetracyclines, it has side-effects. It is now used less frequently than in the past.

Indications
- Acne
- Meningococcal carrier-state prophylaxis.

Dose
- 100 mg to be taken twice a day.

Contraindications
- Children under 12 years of age
- Pregnant/breastfeeding women.

Drug interactions
- With the oral contraceptive pill.

Side-effects
These generally occur if the drug is used for more than 6 months:
- vomiting
- diarrhoea
- skin rash

- light-headedness
- liver damage, therefore a blood test is required every 6 months
- irreversible pigmentation in some patients.

Alternatives
- Topical preparations, such as benzoyl peroxide facial washes
- Antibiotic topical gels, e.g. erythromycin
- Oral preparations, such as erythromycin 500 mg twice a day (however, much bacterial resistance)
- Trimethoprim, 200 mg twice a day
- Oral or topical retinoids (isotretinoin, Roaccutane) – **remember** these are teratogenic and female patients of reproductive age must use adequate contraception.

Discussion

The key point in this scenario is to know about the drug. This patient is under your regular surveillance and you should tell her to come back if she is worried, she also knows what to look out for herself.

If she has been using the drug for longer than 6 months you can offer an alternative treatment. However, if she has only been using minocycline for a short time and has no side-effects, it is probably safe to continue, but you should regularly monitor her for side-effects.

End your discussion with the following:
- 'Is everything clear? Would you like me to repeat anything?'
- 'Do you have any questions for me?'

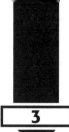

3

Anti-epileptic medication (carbamazepine)

A young woman has recently been diagnosed with epilepsy. Talk to her about her medication.

Answer follows . . .

3

Anti-epileptic medication (carbamazepine)

Answer

Key points

Carbamazepine, trade name Tegretol, is widely used to treat partial seizures and some primary and secondary generalised tonic-clonic seizures. It may also be prescribed for patients with trigeminal neuralgia and as a second-line drug for the prophylaxis of bipolar disorder.

Dose

- Initially, 100 mg carbamazepine is given twice a day for 2 weeks, followed by 200 mg twice a day for a further 2 weeks.
- The dose of carbamazepine may be increased to a maximum of 1 g twice a day.
- A blood test for drug levels may be performed if poor compliance or drug interactions are suspected.

Drug interactions

Patients must be aware that carbamazepine's efficacy may be reduced by its interaction with other drugs, including:

- certain antibiotics, warfarin, diuretics (water tablets), some types of pain relief tablets – therefore the patient should always tell any doctor/chemist that she is taking carbamazepine.
- the oral contraceptive pill – find an alternative method

of contraception
- anti-tuberculous drugs – specifically isoniazid or rifabutin
- alcohol – tell the patient to be cautious of her intake.

Note that the drug may cause photosensitivity, so warn the patient to be careful when sunbathing.

When to contact the doctor
- Any blurring of vision, dizziness or confusion
- Mild reduction in alertness and concentration; this is common, particularly at higher doses
- Altered bowel habits, e.g. diarrhoea/constipation
- Sudden onset of fever with sore throat or a sudden rash
- Sudden onset of mouth ulcers
- Spontaneous or easy bruising
- Bleeding from abnormal sites (e.g. frequent episodes of epistaxis)
- Breast development in males, or new-onset nipple discharge in females.

Discussion

You should advise this patient to take the drug regularly, and as prescribed. Explain that control is based on adequate blood drug levels, and that these may fall to below therapeutic levels if doses are taken very late or skipped.

Suggest she keeps a diary of when the seizures occur, because this is a good indication as to whether the drug/dosage is controlling the epilepsy or if it needs to be altered.

Drugs used post-myocardial infarction

Mr Hart, a 67-year-old man, is an inpatient on CCU. He has been treated for an uncomplicated myocardial infarction and is to be discharged today. You are the SHO working on CCU; please discuss his medications with him.

Answer follows . . .

4

Drugs used post-myocardial infarction

Answer

Remember to introduce yourself to the patient, reassure him that he is making good progress from his heart attack and give him the good news that he is to be discharged today.

If you like, you can start your answer with a definition of a heart attack (see also Chapter 8, Counselling on lifestyle changes after myocardial infarction).

The drugs usually asked about are aspirin, atenolol and GTN. The following are not generally mentioned, but in case they are you can explain that:

- an ACE (angiotensin-converting enzyme) inhibitor helps to strengthen the heart's pumping action
- a statin helps to lower the cholesterol level and reduce the risk of future heart attacks.

You should practise putting the following key points into dialogue.

Key points: low-dose aspirin

Tell the patient the aspirin is to 'thin his blood' and so decrease further blockages of his blood vessels. Explain that it is important to take the tablet with food as otherwise it may irritate the lining of his stomach.

Dose

- One 75-mg tablet to be taken once a day.

Adverse effects

Tell the patient to contact his doctor if he experiences any:

- blackish, tarry, foul-smelling stools (malaena)
- unusual bleeding (e.g. frequent nose bleeds) or excessively bleeding wounds
- shortness of breath or wheeze, particularly if he has a past history of asthma/COPD.

Key points: beta-blockers (e.g. atenolol, trade name Tenormin)

Explain that this tablet helps to prevent the onset of chest pain, or possible 'angina attacks'.

Dose

- One 50-mg tablet to be taken twice a day.

Adverse effects

Tell the patient to contact his doctor if he experiences any:

- dizziness (postural hypotension, bradycardia)
- any shortness of breath or wheeze (bronchospasm)
- very cold hands or feet (peripheral vasoconstriction)
- sleep disturbances, such as nightmares or excessive drowsiness/fatigue in the day
- impotence (there are documented cases of impotence).

Key points: GTN (glyceryl trinitrate, trade names Nitrolingual Pumpspray and Glytrin Spray)

Explain that:

- the drug is taken for the emergency onset of chest pain, or before starting exercises
- it is a good idea to carry this drug with him at all times, in case of emergency
- the tablets are **not** to be swallowed, they will dissolve

under his tongue and be absorbed from there
- he may experience a throbbing headache, but that this side-effect will subside
- facial flushing is also a common side-effect.

Dose
- One 0.5-μg tablet (or 1 or 2 puffs of the spray) is to be used sublingually, as and when needed (i.e. prn, *pro re nata*):
  - repeat if necessary
  - if the pain persists, call for an ambulance.

Adverse effects
Tell the patient to contact his doctor if he experiences any:
- dizziness (postural hypotension)
- increase or worsening chest pain that does not respond to GTN.

Tricyclic antidepressants (TCAs)

Possible case scenarios:

- *Patient needs counselling about using TCAs for the first time.*
- *Patient returning because they feel TCAs aren't helping them.*
- *A patient displaying suicidal intent.*

Answer follows . . .

5

Tricyclic antidepressants (TCAs)

Answer

Key points
Don't forget to introduce yourself. In all cases, adopt an understanding tone, be patient but firm with your response.

Indications
- Depression – particularly endogenous depression requiring sedation
- Other uses – child nocturnal enuresis, trigeminal neuralgia, panic attacks

Drugs
- For example, amitriptyline or dosulepin (dothiepin)

Dose
- Initially, 75 mg single dose to be taken at bedtime.
- Can be increased to 150 mg once a day, or to a maximum of 225 mg once a day (patients on this dose would be hospitalised).

Points to note
However the case is presented to you, some basic ground should be covered in your counselling conversation, bear the following in mind:
- *Is the patient displaying any suicidal intent?*

- You can ask: 'Have you had any ideas about harming yourself? Or planned any ways of ending your life?'
- If the patient genuinely seems to display suicidal intent, it is probably best for you to notify the on-call psychiatrist at the end of your discussion for specialist management.
- *How long has the patient been taking the medication?*
  - Note that TCAs need to be taken for 2–4 weeks before any result will start to show, so the patient must persist with the treatment. It may take 6 weeks before any significant improvement is apparent.
- *Has the patient been taking it regularly?*
  - It is important to check that the right dose is being taken consistently, non-compliance will not benefit the patient.
- *Does the patient insist they have been taking the medication regularly for over a month with no benefit?*
  - You can arrange for a CPN (community psychiatric nurse) to visit the patient and give some extra support.
  - Another alternative is to involve the MHAT (mental health assessment team), a group of community counsellors who can liaise with in-hospital psychiatrists if required.
  - Involving a CPN or MHAT at least ensures some sort of follow-up after the patient leaves your care.

Benefits of the drug
Improved:
- sleep
- appetite
- mood
- sex drive
- concentration.

Once the above are much improved patients can start to help themselves.

Possible side-effects
- Feeling of nausea: an anti-emetic can be prescribed in extreme cases
- Dryness of the mouth: suck on a sweet/on ice/sugar-free sweets
- Urinary retention: in extreme cases patients may present themselves to A&E
- Constipation: can be controlled with diet changes or laxatives
- Blurring of vision/feeling drowsy: avoid driving or operating machinery
- Dizziness on standing: postural hypotension, they should learn to stand in stages, slowly.
  Note that all of the above are anti-muscarinic effects, and the patient should eventually develop a certain tolerance to them.

Less common side-effects
- Arrhythmias
- Convulsions
- Neutropenia (note warning signs of sore throat, fever, rash)
- Galactorrhoea
- Dystonic reaction
- Gynaecomastia.

Discussion

Once you are familiar with the drug and its side-effects you will feel confident in relaying this information to your patient. Practise doing this with a friend/colleague, using the above as a check list.

At the end of all counselling stations remember to ask the following:
- 'Was everything clear for you? Would you like me to repeat anything?'
- 'Do you have any further questions?'

6

Oral contraceptive pills

Any form of contraception is better than none. With any form of contraception, people wish to know how effective yet safe it is, while knowing what side-effects to expect.

You should practise giving the following information in a clear and concise manner. The order in which you give it is important, as there is a lot to say in a small amount of time. An explanation of the contraceptive pill, followed by its advantages, then disadvantages and finally some time for questions at the end is a simple but smart method. Find out what the patient already knows and why they wish to use this method – they may benefit from using an alternative method, such as the male/female condom, intrauterine contraceptive device (IUCD) or depo/injection treatments.

This section will discuss two forms of oral contraceptive: the combined oral contraceptive pill and the progesterone-only pill (the so-called 'mini pill').

Key points

Combined pill

Explain that this pill contains two hormones – oestrogen and progesterone – which are naturally produced and control a woman's monthly cycle. The pill is taken every day for 3 weeks and inhibits ovulation, there is then a pill-free week, during which menstruation can be expected to occur. This method of contraception is very effective. (You should be familiar with the Pearl Index, which gives a typical comparison of pregnancy risk with each form of contraceptive.)

Some long-term advantages include reduced risks of endometrial carcinoma, ovarian carcinoma, endometriosis and pelvic infection. It may also produce lighter, less painful periods. As with any treatment, there are some side-effects. These may include breakthrough bleeding (spotting), headaches, acne and weight gain.

Disadvantages include an increased risk of DVT or MI. Women over 35 years of age are normally not advised to use the combined oral contraceptive pill due to a high risk in thromboembolic disease. It is therefore contraindicated in women with prothrombotic disorders, and in many cardiovascular disorders (varicose veins are not a contraindication). Other contraindications are breast cancer in the patient (or any sex steroid-dependent disease), focal migraine, migraine lasting over 72 hours (status migrainosus), gross obesity and heavy smokers who are over 30 years of age. If the woman is expected to be immobile (e.g. after major surgery), she should stop taking the pill 4 weeks before until 2 weeks after the event and use an alternative method of contraception (e.g. condom) during this time.

Although not a contraindication, the pill must be used with caution in those with a family history of breast cancer, MI, DVT or hypertension. Caution is also required for patients with severe migraine, epilepsy, diabetes or abnormal cervical smears. Rifampicin and anticonvulsant therapy induce liver enzymes thereby reducing the pill's efficacy, so extra precautions are required as ovulation could, in theory, occur. When suffering from diarrhoea or taking antibiotics, extra precautions should be taken during the illness and for 7 days afterwards. Similarly, if a woman forgets to take her pill, she should take it as soon as she remembers, and use precautions for 7 days. If the 7-day period runs into a pill-free week, the next pack should be started without a break. The pill should be stopped at once if unilateral calf pain, breathlessness or other symptoms of

DVT/PE develop. Prolonged headache or severe stomach-ache should also lead her to seek medical advice.

Progesterone-only pill

This pill makes the cervical mucus hostile to sperm. Its advantages over the combined pill are that it can be taken when breast-feeding and most of the oestrogen-dependent contraindications do not apply. It is, however, less effective than the combined pill and can cause erratic bleeding. It must be taken within 3 hours of a set time every day (e.g. 8 am daily), or else extra methods of contraception are needed for 7 days. It is therefore not recommended for women who work shifts.

Switching from the combined pill to the mini-pill, or vice versa, should be accompanied by the use of a condom for the first 7 days. When starting either pill on day 1 of the cycle, contraceptive cover is immediate and no extra precautions are required.

7

The menopause and hormone-replacement therapy (HRT)

Key points

What is the menopause?

The menopause is the cessation of menstruation and can be diagnosed after 1 year's absence of periods. In the UK, the average age of women at the menopause is about 54 years.

Regular menstrual cycles cease because of the decreasing release of ovarian hormones. The onset of the menopause can present with certain symptoms, such as:

- **Early changes** (climacteric or vasomotor changes): hot flushes, irritability, anxiety and forgetfulness, which may progress to vaginal dryness, joint pains and thinning skin
- **Long-term changes**: can result in osteoporosis, heart disease and strokes, the onset of facial hair and balding.

This is where hormone-replacement therapy (HRT) can be used. HRT consists of low-dose oestrogen and progesterones, and has been shown to decrease osteoporosis and possible heart problems after more than 5–10 years' continual use.

Note that HRT is **not** a form of contraception.

HRT preparations

- **Implants**: of oestrogen, which are inserted beneath the skin, and can be used as a depot for up to 6 months. If the uterus is still *in vivo*, oral progesterone is also used for 12 days/month.
- **Patches**: combination patches of oestrogen and

progesterone, which can be used for 2 weeks at a time.

- **Gels:** of oestrogen, which can be rubbed onto the skin (avoiding the breasts) on a daily basis, oral progesterone is prescribed for 12 days/month to women with a uterus.
- **Monthly bleed tablets:** combination of oestrogen and progesterone. These are similar to the oral contraceptive pill, but in low dose. The woman will continue to have regular periods.
- **Three-monthly bleed tablets:** consist of 70 days' oestrogen intake, combined oestrogen and progesterone for 14 days and a placebo for 7 days. This results in four periods per year.
- **Period-free HRT:** continuous HRT tablets. Recommended for women who have been post-menopausal for at least 1 year and are 54 years of age or over.
- **Vaginal preparations:** used topically for urinary symptoms or vaginal dryness; Menoring™, a form of vaginal pessary is now available for systemic menopausal symptoms.

Contraindications

- Liver disease
- Carcinoma of the breast or uterus – breast self-examination encouraged because of the suggested links following a prolonged course of HRT
- Suspicious vaginal bleeding.

Side-effects

- There may be a feeling of breast tenderness and nausea.
- Some women feel bloated.
- Some may get vaginal spotting.

When to contact the doctor

If the patient:
- feels a lump felt in a breast
- has a tender, swollen, painful leg or arm (DVT)
- experiences any irregular bleeding from the vagina.

8

Counselling

Newly diagnosed epilepsy

Miss Fitton, a 22-year-old woman, has recently been diagnosed with epilepsy and is to be discharged today. As the medical house officer on duty, please counsel her about modifications she should make to her lifestyle with regards to her recent diagnosis.

Answer follows . . .

Newly diagnosed epilepsy

Answer

Doctor–patient scenario

Hello Miss Fitton, how are you feeling today? I am Dr M., one of the medical doctors working on the ward. If I may, I would like to talk to you about epilepsy and a few basic things you should be aware of.

To begin with, I would like to explain that epilepsy is a common condition, where there are disturbances in the electrical impulses in the brain. A frequent misconception is that epilepsy is due to an underlying tumour or 'growth' in the brain, this is not true. Also, epilepsy is in no way an infectious condition. Although uncontrolled epilepsy can result in seizures/fits, it is usually very well controlled with medication and you can expect to lead a very normal lifestyle.

However, as epilepsy is a condition where you can have seizures, it is important to take some precautions. For instance, it is always important to eat properly because a sudden drop in your blood sugar may result in a fit, and to sleep properly as you do not want to become overly tired. So it is important to plan time for work and rest.

The mainstay of treatment is your medication, and this must be taken at the correct times and at the correct dose because missing doses will increase your risk of having a seizure.

It would be reassuring to teach people in your home and at

work how to deal with someone having a fit. You may wish to tell your boss discreetly if you don't want all your colleagues to know.

Of course, certain occupations are not compatible with epilepsy, for example drivers, machine operators and other 'at risk' jobs, and you need to discuss this with your boss.

At home, you should initially avoid cooking alone. Similarly, when you're having a shower or a bath try to ensure that someone is nearby, just in case you need help. It may be an idea to get a low bed, rather than a bunk bed for example, to lessen the chances of hurting yourself if you fit during the night.

Very importantly, you must contact the DVLA (Driver and Vehicle Licensing Agency) and inform them about your medical condition. This is for your own safety as well as that of other drivers. As you can imagine, if you sustain a fit when you're driving the results may be catastrophic. I know it sounds very unfair that you must stop driving but this is only a temporary measure until you've been fit-free for a year, after which you can drive again. There are many people with epilepsy who have found a way around the situation.

When you go on holiday always remember to continue to get enough sleep. Avoid too much alcohol as it may trigger a seizure. Be careful with direct exposure to sunlight as it may produce side-effects of your medication (see Carbamazepine, discussed in Chapter 7).

It's also important to keep away from sports such as horse-riding, skiing, parachuting, climbing, etc. Swimming is permissible, but only in shallow waters, and with somebody nearby.

Other triggers of fits can include flashing lights, e.g. the stroboscope at a disco (or in a film), and sitting too close to a computer monitor or TV screen, so keep a reasonable distance away.

Finally, you may wish to purchase a 'Medic-Alert' bracelet. This is an identity bracelet that documents your condition and medication. We recommend these bracelets to people with all sorts of medical conditions, and they can be very useful in case of an emergency. We also suggest that you always carry a list of your medication with you in your purse or pocket.

Well, that's all I would like to tell you before you leave us. I know it was a lot of information in one go, so here's a leaflet containing similar advice to what we've just discussed. As I mentioned earlier, epilepsy is a common condition and there are people who enjoy very normal lives.

Do you have any questions for me?

Thank you for your time Miss Fitton, all the very best in the future.

2

Lifestyle changes advised post-myocardial infarction

Mr Hartwell, a 72-year-old man, is to be discharged today. He was admitted as an inpatient onto a medical ward after suffering an uncomplicated MI. You are the medical SHO. Please explain his condition to him, and advise him about the lifestyle changes he should be thinking about.

Answer follows . . .

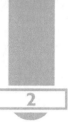

2

Lifestyle changes advised post-myocardial infarction

Answer

Doctor–patient scenario

Hello Mr Hartwell, I'm Dr A., the medical senior house officer. Before you're discharged today I'd like to have a chat with you about your recent heart attack and what you need to do now.

When someone has a heart attack, one of the major vessels in their heart becomes blocked with a clot, this means that the blood (which also contains oxygen) can't circulate to the area of heart which that blood vessel previously supplied. The part of the heart that has been deprived of blood and oxygen is severely injured, and, like any other part of the body, it needs time to rest and recover.

You now need to think about making certain changes to your lifestyle:
- Eat a healthy diet, for example avoid fried fatty foods, cakes, biscuits, etc. to control the cholesterol level in your body. (*Cholesterol can be explained as the 'bad fat in the blood vessels and heart'.*)
- If you smoke, you need to stop completely. You should also reduce your alcohol intake; it's better to cut this out entirely to begin with. (*Explain that tobacco smoke and alcohol are essentially toxins to the body, and that these are risk factors for a heart attack and other medical conditions.*)

- Eat more fruit and vegetables, and especially over the next few months try and include bran in your diet to make sure you don't become constipated; you should avoid straining on the toilet.
- Avoid strenuous activities in general.
- Avoid driving over the next month.
- We strongly advise patients who have had a heart attack to rest when they are discharged, but this doesn't simply mean bed rest. (*If the patient still goes out to work, they should take time off – a sick note may be issued if necessary.*)
- However, you should take up a gentle form of regular exercise, like walking, but nothing that makes you out of breath, or brings on chest pain (this can include vigorous sexual activity).
- You should take your medications regularly for the heart attack, and any other medications you are taking. This is because your heart has become a little weaker and if another medical condition becomes very bad then your heart may be affected again.
- A follow-up appointment will be made for 6 weeks' time. An exercise tolerance test/treadmill test may then be carried out to see how well your heart is healing from the recent injury.
- Most patients are referred for cardiac rehabilitation – this is a programme of exercise and education, someone will get in touch with you to give you the details.
- I know this has been rather a lot to take in, is there anything you want me to go over again? Are there any questions you'd like to ask me?
- Thank you, Mr Hartwell, and all the best.

Panic attacks

Imagine you are an SHO working in the psychiatry outpatient department. A 32-year-old woman, Miss Fretting, comes to your clinic as a GP referral. She has been diagnosed as suffering from panic attacks. How would you manage this situation?

Answer follows . . .

3

Panic attacks

Answer

This is an easy scenario to lose track of and you can become side-tracked onto non-relevant issues. It is important to keep a check-list of key points in mind and to cover the following:

- What could be the trigger for the panic attacks?
- Are there any symptoms of depression?
- Are there any signs of self-harm/suicidal intent?
- Rule out organic causes.
- Get a general social picture to aid further management plans.

Doctor-patient scenario

DR M.: Good morning Miss Fretting, I'm very pleased to meet you, my name is Dr M. and I'm the SHO.

MISS F.: Hello Dr M.

DR M.: Could you tell me what seems to be the problem, and what brought you here today?

MISS F.: I don't really know doctor, all I know is that I'm not coping very well at present, and my GP has made an appointment for me.

DR M.: Your GP seems to think that you are worrying too much about a lot of things, is that correct? Are there any things in particular?

MISS F.: Well, I don't really know where to start, I mean I wasn't always like this, it just seems to be . . . well, recently. I don't know what's happening to me.

DR M.: When do you usually get worried and how do you feel at the time?

MISS F.: It seems to be more and more frequent these days, even small things will set me off – like forgetting to buy something at the supermarket. I start to feel dizzy and short of breath. It's a truly horrible feeling, I think I'm going to die.

(*Here is your cue, the actress isn't going to give you any more specific information. You need to start ruling things out, so start asking questions.*)

1. How long have you been getting worried like this? Was anything else happening in your life at the time?
   - Determining the onset of these symptoms may give you an idea of any major life events that could trigger such behaviour – look out for divorce, separation, bereavement, miscarriage, loss of a job, etc.
2. If she doesn't give a definite answer to Question 1, try to establish a cause:
   - Are there any problems of stress at work or at home?
   - Do you have a partner? Is he supportive?
   - What do you do for a living?
   - Do you have any children? How are they?
   - Are you having any financial problems? Or housing problems?
   - How do you cope with your daily activities, do you go out? Do you have a group of friends?
3. Think about medical causes, rule out:
   - **Hyperthyroidism**: How are you in yourself, your periods? Your bowels? Your appetite/weight? Do you have a particular dislike for hot weather? Do you notice you are more shaky/sweaty than usual?
   - **Depression**: Are you ever able to stop worrying and relax? Do you sleep well? How is your appetite? Do you feel tired or lethargic? Are you able to concentrate?
   - **Obsessive–compulsive disorder**: Have you noticed

that you've started doing certain things repeatedly, for example washing your hands or checking the front door lock?
- ○ **Family history**: Has anyone in your family suffered with any psychiatric illness?
- ○ **Side-effects**: Are you on any medications, either ones your doctor has prescribed or you've bought over the counter?'

4. Have you ever tried to harm yourself or anyone else as a result of not being able to cope? Do you think you might attempt this again?
- ○ If self-harm or suicidal ideation is displayed then follow the 'Depression management plan' with a community psychiatric nurse, antidepressants (see TCAs in Chapter 7). Inpatient management may be required.

5. Social history:
- ○ Do you drink or smoke? How much? What do you drink?
- ○ Do you take any recreational drugs? What do you take? How much?

Obviously, if any one of the above becomes apparent early on in the discussion you must confirm your diagnosis and follow an appropriate management plan.

Differential diagnoses

For this station, think about the following differential diagnoses:
- drug withdrawal
- alcoholism
- obsessive–compulsive disorder
- hyperthyroidism
- depression
- family history of psychiatric illness
- side-effects of medications
- drug abuse, e.g. LSD, cocaine, amphetamines.

Management

Panic attacks in general are managed by:

- identifying and stopping the offending factor
- using a brown paper bag to re-breathe into (avoids hyperventilation)
- practising relaxation techniques
- prescribing cognitive-behavioural therapy
- trying benzodiazepines; these may help in the short term
- consider an SSRI such as Citalopram or Paroxetine.

4

Ovarian cyst

A 35-year-old woman has been diagnosed with an ovarian cyst on the right side. On ultrasound, the cyst is 8.5 cm in diameter. A decision to perform right ovarian cystectomy has been made. Explain the condition to her and obtain her informed consent. She is expected to remain in the hospital for 5 days after the operation, and the surgeon concerned will be using a suprapubic incision and a subcuticular wound closure using a fine prolene suture material. Explain that 6 weeks' restricted activity is normally advised after such a procedure.

Answer follows . . .

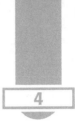

4

Ovarian cyst

Answer

Key points

Practise putting the following points into dialogue.

Start by greeting the patient and introducing yourself.

While explaining her condition try to avoid using as much medical terminology as possible, but don't patronise the patient. Inform her that the scan showed a cyst, which is a fluid-filled swelling, measuring 8.5 cm in diameter on her right ovary. She might be alarmed by this information and may ask you to explain its significance. As the type of proposed surgery is stated in the question, it is reasonable to assume the cyst is benign, otherwise more information would have been given. Therefore you can reassure the patient by saying that in all probability the cyst is not cancerous. You can then tell her that the cyst needs to be the removed. Now proceed to explain what right ovarian cystectomy means. Say that to remove this cyst from her right ovary, we will have to cut open her tummy by making an incision just above her pubic hairline. During surgery, the cyst will be removed while conserving the ovary. We will then close the different layers of her tummy and suture the skin incision using a non-absorbable thread. Inform her that the method of suturing her skin is by subcuticular closure, which means the thread runs underneath the skin. Tell the patient that because it is non-absorbable, the suture will need to be removed 5 days later.

While obtaining the patient's consent it is vitally important that her correct name, date of birth and hospital number are written on the consent form, together with mention of the correct site of operation is mentioned. During your consultation you must address all the patient's fears and worries regarding the surgery. If she asks you questions that are your beyond your level of knowledge, it is always wise to tell her that you will ask your consultant or any other senior member of the team to speak to her in this regard. You **must not** provide wrong information. Seek help from your seniors when you are unsure about anything. The new adult consent form, now used universally in the UK, requires you to make the patient aware of the complications of the surgery, the need for blood transfusion and any additional procedure that might become necessary to deal with complications arising from the primary surgery. For example, if you are consenting a patient for myomectomy it is prudent to consent her for a hysterectomy. If the patient refuses to sign the consent form then you need to seek senior help, and in such cases the surgery may be deferred or cancelled.

You must counsel the woman with the ovarian cyst about complications such as bleeding, infection and perforation to the bladder, bowel, blood vessels and other nearby organs. Since this is a major pelvic surgical procedure, it is also important that she is made aware of the risk of developing a clot in her lungs or limbs (i.e. PE and DVT). Make sure you do not over-alarm the patient when talking about these complications, instead reassure her that the chance of these complications occurring are extremely remote. The universal complication figure quoted for all surgeries is 1 in 1000. As this is an informed consent, you are duty bound to inform the patient of all the risks associated with the surgery. While consenting this woman you also have to obtain her consent for additional procedures, such as oophorectomy and the repair of any organ damage. The cyst is a fairly large one and if it is too distorted then it might be difficult to preserve the ovary, so consenting her for a right oophorectomy is wise. It is important to reassure her at this stage that if she wishes to have children in the future then this surgery should not affect her chances of becoming pregnant in any way. You must also ensure she is aware of the remote possibility of the need for a blood transfusion.

Complete your discussion by telling her that the operation is going to be done under general anaesthesia; that when she regains consciousness in the recovery room she might feel groggy and find tubes running through her veins providing intravenous fluids and a catheter draining her bladder. You can also tell her that to reduce the risk of developing a clot in her lungs or legs she will be given blood-thinning injections subcutaneously, once a day, during her stay in the hospital. While talking about her post-operative stay in hospital you can inform her that the catheter and the tubes providing iv fluids usually come out after 24–36 hours, and if all is fine she will be discharged after about 5 days. On discharge, tell her that she needs to maintain 6 weeks of restricted activity, and she will be reviewed in the clinic at that time to discuss her future follow-up.

The patient may ask you when they can start driving again. It is reasonable to assume they can start driving once they resume their normal activities. However, if in doubt ask the DVLA, Swansea, for advice in this regard.

End your conversation by wishing the patient all the best for the surgery and for a speedy recovery.

5

Sexually transmitted infection

A 22-year-old patient presents to you complaining of a smelly genital discharge. What would you say to this patient?

Answer follows . . .

5

Sexually transmitted infection

Answer

Key points

(See also 'Vaginal discharge' in Chapter 2.)

Today, sexually transmitted infections (STIs) comprise one of the most important groups of infectious diseases, and lead to high morbidity among the young adult population of this country. The most important sexually transmitted diseases (STDs) are chlamydia, gonorrhoea, genital herpes, genital warts, *Trichomonas vaginalis* infection, syphilis, human immunodeficiency virus (HIV) infection and bacterial vaginosis. In recent years there has been a marked increase in the number of cases of chlamydia and gonorrhoea.

Symptoms

The presenting symptoms in the acute phase of any of the STDs are very similar. Most female patients usually complain of a smelly, itchy and mucopurulent vaginal discharge. Associated symptoms may include pelvic pain and tenderness, dyspareunia and bleeding irregularities, such as post-coital bleeding, intermenstrual bleeding or breakthrough bleeding while on the contraceptive pill (it is worth mentioning here that the young contraceptive-pill taker is most at risk of contracting a sexually transmitted diseases). Persistent genital swelling or non-healing genital or oral ulcers may also feature at presentation. However, the picture is becoming increasingly complex in people infected with HIV: here the presenting features are more commonly caused by atypical secondary infections, such as pneumocystis pneumonia or incurable persistent oral candidiasis.

Male patients suffer from a smelly and itchy urethral discharge, genital ulcers or warts. Whereas, proctitis, rectal discharge, rectal bleeding and rectal warts and ulcers can occur in homosexuals.

Complications

Pelvic inflammatory diseases (PIDs), including salpingitis, cervicitis and tubo-ovarian abscesses, are a sequel of STIs in the female population. Moreover, subfertility, ectopic pregnancies and chronic pelvic pain are long-term complications of STDs in women, while subfertility may be transient or permanent in men. Recurrent cystitis and urinary tract infections (UTIs) occur in both the sexes but are more common in females.

Screening for STIs

Previously, enzyme-linked immunosorbent assays (ELISA) were used to check for these infections, but now more sophisticated tests, such as the PCR technique (polymerase chain reaction), are commonly being used, which give a significantly lower number of false-positive results.

It is important to screen for STIs in all women undergoing termination of pregnancy, a significant number of whom usually test positive. Similarly, all women attending family planning clinics for insertion of intrauterine contraceptive devices (IUCDs) should be screened for STIs; again these women are at high risk of contracting STIs.

High-vaginal swabs and endocervical swabs are taken to test for chlamydia, bacterial vaginosis and gonorrhoea in women, while urethral swabs are taken in men. A first-void urine sample can also be used to test for chlamydial and gonococcal infections. All ulcers caused by STIs need to be swabbed and tested. Rectal swabs are taken mainly in the homosexual male population. Blood serology is used to test for most of the other STIs.

Follow-up

This will depend on the results of the various tests. All patients who test positive for an STI need to be urgently referred to the genitourinary medicine (GUM) clinic for follow-up and contact tracing. Contact tracing is a vital tool in containing the spread of these infections.

Doctor–patient scenario

Practise putting the following into dialogue.

Taking a history for STIs may prove to be tricky due to the associated social stigma. It is, therefore, important to ask direct questions, while at the same time reassuring the patient that any information will be treated with the utmost confidence.

Start by asking if the patient is sexually active or not. It is important to remember that if you are seeing a young girl who is not yet sexually active, you should rule out STIs straight away and not subject her to any examination. While taking a history for STIs it is necessary to know if the patient is in a stable relationship (monogamous) or has had a number of different relationships in recent months (polygamous). You may also ask if the patient is in a homosexual or heterosexual relationship, as the disease prevalence is different in these two groups. While the incidence of HIV is in decline in the homosexual male population, it is increasing at alarming proportions in the heterosexual population.

Proceed to ask about the symptoms mentioned above. It is

also helpful to ask if their partner(s) suffers from the same symptoms, which may help in contact tracing. Also ask about drug use and social circumstances – the increase in the number of STIs among drug abusers is primarily caused by sharing infected needles, and a high incidence of STIs has also been reported among members of poor socioeconomic groups.

Tell the patient that you would like to take some samples for testing (remember to ask their permission) and what a positive result will mean for their follow-up. You should also counsel the patient about the need to avoid infecting other people.

Don't forget to end by thanking the patient for their co-operation.

6

Breaking bad news – diagnosis of cancer

You are the SHO in a breast clinic. Discuss the diagnosis of cancer with this patient.

Answer follows . . .

6

Breaking bad news – diagnosis of cancer

Answer

This is a skill that transcends all areas of medicine. We will use breast cancer as an example of a potential OSCE station, but the method is the same for any type of bad news. While this section will concentrate on the approach to this scenario, an in-depth understanding of the condition involved and the patient's history is imperative in real-life situations as you will otherwise struggle to answer their questions, and similarly may ask insensitive questions about their past in the process.

SPIKES* – a protocol for breaking bad news

This mnemonic refers to the stages involved in breaking bad news.

S – The setting

Before the interview begins, take some time to create an appropriate environment. For example, make sure your bleep won't disturb you and that you have sufficient time to break the news. Ensure privacy by closing doors or curtains. Avoid having a barrier (e.g. a desk) between you and the patient and make good use of your history-taking skills (good eye contact, empathy, appropriate silences and listening, clear explanations with little jargon; use open

*SPIKES was devised by Dr Walter Baile and Dr Robert Buckman.

questions when beginning to allow the patient to talk freely). You may wish to have a nurse present who can answer questions later if you are unavailable. Ask the patient if they would like anyone else (friend, relative) to be present.

P – Patient's perception

When you start talking, find out what the patient already knows or believes about their condition, what their concerns are, and what they expect will happen immediately/in the future. A useful way of remembering this step is to use the mnemonic **ICE**:

- Ideas
- Concerns
- Expectations.

I – Invitation

Find out how much the patient wants to know. This is also a good way of preparing the patient for the coming bad news; for example, by asking: 'Are you the sort of person who wants to know everything about their condition?' This technique is known as a 'warning shot'.

K – Knowledge

This is the step in which you break the bad news, and the one that probably needs the most sensitivity on your part. How much you tell them depends on what they told you in step 'I', and how they react as they begin to hear your news. This is where your knowledge is also important, but remember to avoid using confusing terms. Do not give false reassurances. Give any information in small segments, and make sure they understand everything you tell them before moving on.

E – Explore emotions and empathise

You need to be prepared for their reaction, whatever it may be. Some people may be shocked and become silent, while others may refuse to believe you and get angry. You should try to explore why they feel the way they do. You may already understand why from their ICE (step P in SPIKES). You should also reassure them that their reaction is understandable under the circumstances. When the news comes as a total shock it may be necessary to explore ICE again.

S – Strategy and summary

Don't leave a patient feeling uncertain about the next step after the interview – summarise what you discussed and suggest a strategy for the immediate future. For example, if further tests are needed then explain what they will involve and when they may be done. Remember even a patient beyond medical treatment can still be told about palliative care, and can be assured that they can live out the rest of their days with dignity and support. Terminal patients may have concerns about what will happen to their loved ones after they die – you can also discuss things like finances and wills if appropriate, though this is best left for a later discussion.

Doctor–patient scenario

The following scenario uses the steps discussed above.

S – The setting

(*This has been discussed above. Good communication skills will be shown throughout the dialogue that follows.*)

P – Patient perception

DR M.: Hello Mrs B., thank you for coming in. Sorry for the wait. Did your husband not come with you this time?

MRS B.: Yes, he said he'll be along soon.

DR M.: Would you like to wait for him?

MRS B.: No, that's quite alright, he said to go on without him.

DR M.: Do take a seat. How are you feeling?

MRS B.: I feel fine.

DR M.: Good. I understand you were referred by your GP. Did you know why you were sent here?

MRS B.: I found a lump in my right breast a few weeks ago so I went to my GP for him to have a look at it. After he'd examined it he said I'd need to come in for some tests.

DR M.: Okay. What did you think the lump was – did you have any concerns about the lump?

MRS B.: Obviously, the first thing that comes to your mind is cancer.

DR M.: What made you think of cancer?

MRS B.: My mother had breast cancer before she died and I know it sometimes runs in families, so I was a little worried.

DR M.: So is that why you went to your GP?

MRS B.: Yes.

I – Invitation

DR M.: You had some tests for the lump last time you were in clinic. Is that right?

MRS B.: That's right. Have the results come back yet?

DR M.: Yes they have. I actually have them in front of me now. Would you like to know the result now – or do you want to bring your husband in?

MRS B.: Is it bad news?

DR M.: It's not quite what we were hoping for . . . do you want me to carry on?

MRS B.: Yes, I'm not sure if my husband would want to hear this.

DR M.: If you want him to join us at any time just say.

K – Knowledge

DR M.: Some of the cells we took last time to look at under the microscope came back as abnormal.

MRS B.: Abnormal?

DR M.: Yes. They showed changes that are cancerous.

(*You pause to see how she reacts to this. Mrs B. doesn't say anything for a few seconds, during which time you decide not to rush her.*)

MRS B.: I see. What's going to happen now?

DR M.: It looks like the lump in your breast is a cancer. However, because it's quite small we don't think it has spread anywhere else. To be sure, we'd like to do some more tests.

MRS B.: What tests?

DR M.: We'd like to take some special X-rays of your chest in something we call a CT scanner – have you heard of that?

MRS B.: Yes, they did one on my father after he had a stroke.

DR M.: After that we would remove the lump by doing an operation.

E – Explore emotions and empathise

DR M.: Do you understand everything I've told you so far?

MRS B.: Yes I think so. I had thought about cancer, but it's a shock when you hear it.

DR M.: How are you feeling now?

MRS B.: I don't know. I'm wondering what's going to happen to me.

DR M.: How do you mean?

MRS B.: I'm scared that what happened to my mother will happen to me.

DR M.: That's perfectly understandable, but remember that we've found this cancer very early on, so there's a good chance we'll be able to treat it successfully. Is there anything else worrying you?

MRS B.: I've not really had time to think about it. Will I have to lose my breast?

DR M.: It's hard to say at the moment, but it may be necessary. If that was the case it could still be possible to reconstruct your breast. I know it's a lot to think about right now . . .

S – Strategy and summary

. . . but you can ask as many questions as you like whenever you want. You don't have to ask everything now – you can come back to see me, or phone the nurses at any time.

MRS B.: Thank you. I might have to do that.

DR M.: Okay, is there anything else you want to ask now?

MRS B.: I can't think of anything.

DR M.: That's fine. I'll start to arrange the CT scan now, and we'll contact you at home when you need to come in. I think the operation will be quite soon after that – maybe by the end of the month. Take care, see you soon.

7

Emergency contraception

Ms Jackson is 14 years old and claims her ex-boyfriend has raped her. She presents to you in A&E with a police escort. Unprotected sex occurred about 72 hours ago.

Answer follows . . .

7

Emergency contraception

Answer

Key points

Once again, this is a difficult question, having a number of issues that need to be addressed. First, it is important to understand that this is a medico-legal case as the patient is a minor and she has been raped. The main issues here are the medico-legal aspect of the case and the establishment of Frasier Guidelines (formerly known as Gillick competence). It is important to establish at the outset whether the boyfriend is an adult or also a minor, as the law will be different in the two cases. However, as the A&E doctor you are expected to examine, treat and advise the patient in the best possible way in such distressing circumstances. The police surgeon deals with most of the medico-legal aspects. Practise putting the following points into dialogue.

Start by introducing yourself and offering her sympathy and reassurance. It is important to take the patient's verbal consent before proceeding with any intimate gynaecological examination, as she could be still quite shocked from her traumatic experience. It is also important to establish Frasier Guidelines in the very beginning. In brief, Frasier Guidelines state that a minor has the right to decide and consent to any medical treatment provided to her, without parental consent irrespective of her age, if it is found that she has the mental maturity and understanding to do so. Once that is established, proceed to offer her all the screening tests for sexually transmitted diseases. While examining the patient (**in the presence of a chaperone**) look for inspectory findings suggestive of forceful penetration. Look for any signs of trauma, bruising, laceration and haematoma on the external genitalia, breasts and other parts of the body. If she is a virgin, look for a torn hymen and other signs of resistance, e.g. bruising along the inner folds of the groin.

Another important aspect in this case is to discuss emergency contraception with the patient. It is important to know when the intercourse took place to be able to provide the best emergency contraception in such circumstances. In this case it was 72 h ago. Essentially, there are two methods of emergency contraception: levonorgestrol and the IUD. Emergency contraceptive pills must be taken within 72 hours of having unprotected sex, but are more effective the sooner they are taken. There are two different types of hormonal emergency pills: the progesterone-only pill (POP; levonorgestrol) – a pack of two pills; and the combined oral contraceptive – a pack of four pills (Yuzpe regimen). Both are taken in the same way: the first dose (one pill in the case of POP, and two in the Yuzpe regimen) is taken as soon as possible after unprotected sex, followed 12 h later by the second dose. The most commonly used regimen is levonorgestrol 75 mg in two doses 12 h apart. The pills act by preventing ovulation, delaying ovulation and preventing implantation. Emergency contraceptive pills are very effective if taken immediately after unprotected intercourse and prevent four out of five pregnancies. They are most likely to fail if taken after 72 hours; if the patient vomits within 3 hours of taking the pill; if she forgets to take the second pill; or if she has had unprotected sex at another time since her last period or since taking the emergency pill. The patient should have a period within 3 weeks of taking the emergency contraceptive (EC); if she doesn't, then a pregnancy test should be performed.

Another EC option, still on trial, is mifepristone. This anti-progesterone, taken up to 5 days following unprotected intercourse, prevents 80% of expected pregnancies. It is effective in a wide range of doses, the lowest being 10 mg. The higher the dose the more likely it is that menses are postponed, because one of the mechanisms of action is to delay ovulation. However, even at low doses there are availability and cost problems.

If it is too late for the patient to take emergency pills (over 72 hours since unprotected intercourse), does not or cannot take hormones, wants to use the most effective method of emergency contraception or wants the IUD as a long-term method, then the best contraceptive is the copper IUD. It can be fitted within 5 days of having unprotected intercourse or within 5 days of the last ovulation. However, the IUD is not suitable for all women. If the patient is at risk of contracting a sexually transmitted infection (by having more then one partner or her partner having other partners), she could develop a pelvic infection. It is advisable to perform screening tests at the time the IUD is fitted and to give some antibiotics to prevent a pelvic infection. The copper IUD is 100% effective. It acts by preventing the egg from being fertilised or implanted in the womb although it does not prevent ectopic pregnancy.

In this case scenario, the IUD looks to be the best option. Once the IUD has been fitted remind the patient to see her GP or nurse in 3/4 weeks' time for a check-up to make sure she is not pregnant. The IUD can be removed during her next period if she doesn't want to use the IUD as a long-term contraceptive method.

Once you have covered all these issues with the patient, end your conversation by thanking her for her co-operation.

8

Tubal sterilisation

Ms Grant is a 26-year-old woman who would like to be sterilised, she is a career woman, and does not feel that she would want children in the future. Explain tubal sterilisation to her and decide if she should go ahead with the procedure or not.

Answer follows . . .

Tubal sterilisation

Answer

Key points

Practise putting the following points into dialogue.

Greet the patient and introduce yourself to her.

This is an extremely tricky situation, as here you have a young woman with no children requesting sterilisation. The issues that need to be discussed are whether she is absolutely certain of her decision, whether she has exhausted all the other long-term reversible contraceptive methods and whether she realises the irreversibility of the procedure. Usually in such situations the patient is absolutely adamant that she wants to be sterilised.

First establish whether she is in a stable relationship. If she says 'Yes', then try and counsel her about the long-term reversible contraceptive methods, such as implants, injections and intrauterine contraceptive devices, which can give her contraceptive cover with high efficacy for 6 months, 3 years and 5 years. You can also counsel her about her partner opting to have a vasectomy. However, if she is not in a stable relationship you can counsel her about the risk of changing personal circumstances in the future when she might want to raise a family. Hence, as tubal sterilisation is, to all intents, an irreversible procedure having extremely low success rates when reversed, the only way to achieve pregnancy in such circumstances would be to opt for IVF. Stress the fact that it is an extremely important decision she is making which might have future consequences. It would be wise to involve a consultant at this stage. However, if she is still steadfast in her decision then, after carefully documenting all your discussion in the notes, proceed to talk about the surgery. At the end of the day, you have to respect the patient's decision.

Explain to the patient how tubal sterilisation is performed. We are talking about laparoscopic sterilisation where a cut is made in the patient's belly button and a telescopic camera is used to perform the surgery. Another small cut is made in the suprapubic region to allow entry of the instrument. Both tubes are identified and ligation clips are applied near the isthmic end of the tubes to prevent fertilisation. Usually the procedure is done as a day-case procedure and if all is fine the patient is discharged the same day. Since the operation is performed under general anaesthesia, a responsible adult should be there to take the patient home and look after her for the next 48 hours. Although the operation is classified as a minor laparoscopic procedure, it is important to counsel the patient about the associated risk of surgical complications, i.e. bleeding, perforation and infection. In the unlikely circumstance of organ damage, it is important to make the patient aware that a laparotomy (which means a wider cut just above the pubic hair line) will be performed to repair the damage. If that happens, her stay in the hospital would increase and so would the morbidity from the surgery. Once again, make sure you do not unnecessarily alarm the patient by stating the risks of the procedure, but reassure her by saying that there is a low probability of this happening.

While counselling about sterilisation you have to talk about the failure rate being 1 in 200, which means there is a 1 in 200 chance that she will become pregnant even after sterilisation. You also need to make her aware that in the unlikely scenario that she does conceive after sterilisation there is an increased risk of her having an ectopic pregnancy. Inform her that the procedure is best done immediately after a period.

End your discussion by thanking the patient and telling her that, since this an elective procedure, she could still take time to think over her decision before finally deciding to go ahead.

9

Antenatal genetic counselling – Down's syndrome

You are the SHO working in an obstetrics and gynaecology clinic. A 35-year-old woman, Mrs D., presents to you for the results of her triple test. The results show there is a high probability that her child has Down's syndrome. Please counsel her about the test results.

Answer follows . . .

9

Antenatal genetic counselling – Down's syndrome

Answer

We shall use Down's syndrome as an example of a genetic disorder that can be detected antenatally. The aims of counselling are to give information on chromosomal/congenital diseases, which may or may not present at birth but could potentially affect the child's quality of life. It is important to discuss how the condition will affect the child's life (should it occur), what the risk factors and calculated risks are for acquiring it and what treatment and support is necessary. It is important to make sure all information is understood – for example, the risk of two carrier parents having a baby with cystic fibrosis is 1 in 4, but some parents may think this means they will have three unaffected children before having one affected child, which may not be the case. All information must be given in an unbiased way, and the parents must be given the time and autonomy to make their own choice about how to proceed.

Key points

Investigations

Screening for Down's syndrome is offered to all pregnant women at the booking scan around the twelfth week of pregnancy. Risk factors include a history of Down's syndrome in a previous child (6% of cases of Down's syndrome results from a Robertsonian translocation between chromosomes 14 and 21), increased maternal age >35 years and the results of the triple test and ultrasound scan. The triple test measures levels of maternal serum alpha-fetoprotein, human chorionic gonadotrophin and oestriol, and gives a risk of developing the condition. The ultrasound scan measures nuchal translucency (assessing the skin fold thickness of the back of the neck). Both the triple test and nuchal translucency are screening tests at 10–14 weeks' gestation. The results of the triple test, ultrasound scan and the risk associated with maternal age (see Table 8.1) are combined to give an overall risk; but is still not a definitive diagnosis of Down's syndrome.

Table 8.1 Risk of having a Down's syndrome affected child with increasing maternal age

Maternal age (years)	Risk
20	1/1700
25	1/1400
30	1/900
35	1/400
40	1/100
45	1/35

Women with high-risk pregnancies are offered chorionic villous sampling (CVS) or amniocentesis. Both these karyotyping techniques are very sensitive (they detect the majority of affected babies). Although the results of CVS are available in 24–48 h (amniocentesis takes 2–3 weeks), the miscarriage rate following CVS is slightly higher than with amniocentesis (for which it is 1%). In some advanced centres a recent technique known as FISH (Fluorescent ImmunoSorbent Hylondisation technique) can give a result within 5 days, from the amniocentesis.

Discussing the results with the parents

Be prepared for emotional responses from both parents when giving them potentially bad news. If possible, both parents should be present. It is important to be sensitive at all times, allowing time for questions and stressing that antenatal care is ongoing and that they can receive further advice and help at any time. Before explaining a high-risk result it is advisable to gauge the parents' understanding of the condition.

Doctor–patient scenario

You may find the following role-play useful for OSCE situations:

DR M.: Hello Mr and Mrs D., I'm Dr M.

MR and MRS D.: Hello.

DR M.: I understand you took a test recently to assess the risk of Down's syndrome in your baby. Can I ask what you understand by the term Down's syndrome?

MRS D.: We know it's a genetic thing that causes learning difficulties in children. Is that right?

DR M.: Yes that's right. It is genetic and it can cause developmental problems as well as other problems in children. Do you understand what happens in the genes to cause the condition?

MRS D.: Not really. I don't really know at all – can you explain how it occurs?

DR M.: Yes of course. Think of every cell in your body having information inside it, coding for everything: one bit codes for the colour of your eyes, while another bit may code for how curly your hair will be. All these codes are something we call DNA and this DNA is arranged into long strings of information called chromosomes. Every human usually has 23 pairs of chromosomes. When a mother has a baby, she passes on one copy of her chromosomes to the baby and the father passes on one copy of his chromosomes, so that the baby receives an equal amount of DNA from each parent, and like them, ends up with 23 pairs of chromosomes. However, in most cases of Down's syndrome, one parent passes on two copies of the 21st chromosome and so the baby ends up with three copies of it. We can calculate if a mother has a high risk of having a child with Down's syndrome through the blood test you had recently. However, the result of the test is only a risk – so a person with a high risk does not necessarily have a baby with Down's syndrome – in fact, a high risk is considered to be a 1 in 200 chance. The risk gets higher as the mother gets older, but a 20-year-old mum with a risk of 1 in 1700 can still give birth to an affected child – it's only a risk – not a diagnosis – do you see what I mean?

MRS D.: Yes. Do you have my results?

DR M.: Yes, they came through today. Would you like to know the result now?

MRS D.: Is it bad news?

DR M.: You have to remember it's not a diagnosis, but the result showed you to be in what we consider the high-risk category.

(Silence)

MRS D.: But this doesn't mean my child has Down's, does it?

DR M.: No, but we can give you a more definite result either way if we do some further tests.

MRS D.: Okay. What tests?

Although terminations can occur up to 24 weeks (and in some cases, any time before birth), this may not always be the most desirable course of action. With modern standards of medical care, Down's children can lead very happy and loving lives, well into their mid-forties. It is up to you to make sure the mother and family have the information and support needed to make her own decision. Always allow time for the family to ask questions either at the consultation or afterwards. Also, stress the availability of information from support groups such as the Down's Syndrome Association.

10

Post-natal counselling – cerebral palsy

Suppose you were the SHO who had discovered certain abnormalities in the neonatal check suggestive of cerebral palsy – how would you tell the parents?

Answer follows . . .

10

Post-natal counselling – cerebral palsy

Answer

While Down's syndrome can be screened for antenatally, cerebral palsy (CP) may only become apparent during the neonatal period, because this is a condition characterised by a lesion to the brain acquired around the time of birth (before, during or after). The first time it may be diagnosed could be at the neonatal check performed by the paediatrician, or even later in the GP setting. CP has no cure, and can result in significant developmental delay. This section deals with how to counsel an affected child's parents with due sensitivity and empathy, as with antenatal counselling. You should also be familiar with the 'Breaking bad news' section elsewhere in this chapter.

Key points

- Ensure a suitable undisturbed setting where you can talk to both the parents and relatives in private.
- Introduce yourself to the family and have a nurse present, if possible, who will be able to answer any questions after you have left, and would be a witness to everything you say.
- Explain that you are the SHO and have performed a post-natal check on their baby (use the baby's name if possible). Say you've found some things that you'd like to discuss with them. This would be a good way of assessing their reaction to what you are about to say (this

technique is known as a 'warning shot').

- Depending on their reaction, go on to say you'd found certain features on their baby that may suggest a condition known as cerebral palsy. (*There is little point in beating around the bush, as you have a lot of material to discuss with the parents. However, every parent is different, and not all will be ready for such a direct approach.*)
- Neonatally, these features could be facial features – including: a small head circumference; symptomatic hypoglycaemia/seizures; abnormal neurological signs; and possible increased muscle tone and/or abnormal movements. Obviously, explain findings relevant to their child in a way the parents will understand.
- Go on to explain how this condition occurs, that CP is due to a lesion in the brain occurring around the time of birth, it is not a genetic condition and is hard to diagnose antenatally. If, as happens in some cases, it was due to a unavoidable traumatic birth, explain the difficulties experienced during the delivery. Have your consultant present if there are legal implications for the hospital.

Having established the child is likely to be affected, most parents will want to know exactly how disabling the condition will be. You may be able to give a rough indication from your examination findings, but remember all you have is a snapshot of that child, and while the condition is non-progressive, it is not unchanging. Similarly, while there is no cure, it can be treated. It is important to gauge how much the parents want to hear at this stage, and you should stress the fact that they can receive further help and consultations at any time. Many parents may be too shocked to continue as all their expectations for a 'normal' child are shattered. However, depending on the area of brain affected, possible presentations include:

○ learning difficulties: 60% (although many have

normal intelligence)
- o epilepsy: 40%
- o squint: 30%
- o visual impairment: 20%
- o speech and language disorders due to problems with muscles, learning and hearing
- o spasticity: affects over 70% of those with CP, leading to reduced function of one arm and leg (hemiparesis), legs affected more than arms (diplegia), or even all limbs affected (quadriparesis).

- Tell the parents that their child might have delayed motor milestones, an abnormal gait once they begin to walk, feeding difficulties and developmental delay with language and social skills.
- Because all this would be a lot for any mother or father to take on board, mention that their child will have ongoing treatment from a multidisciplinary team which includes paediatricians, speech therapists, physiotherapists, occupational therapists and so on. For example: paediatricians will help to monitor their child's development; speech therapists can help mothers with feeding early on; physiotherapists can make sure a child reaches their full potential physically, occupational therapists may suggest improvements in the house to decrease handicap.
- Mention that each child with CP will still achieve the realistic goals set for them, and that everything will be done to help maximise their child's chances of reaching their full potential in all aspects of life.
- Ask them if they have any questions and possibly arrange for them to spend some time with the nurse, if present, as well as making a follow-up appointment with yourself or your consultant.
- Finally, thank the parents.

11

Post-natal depression

Mrs John is a 28-year-old woman who delivered her baby 2 months ago. She is not coping well at home. She presents to you in outpatients with her husband, who feels she is not bonding with the baby. Mrs John is tearful and clearly distressed. Please ask relevant questions and counsel her.

Answer follows . . .

11

Post-natal depression

Answer

Psychiatric problems related to pregnancy include:

- **Baby blues**: These are usually mild and resolve fairly quickly (2–3 weeks) and spontaneously, with a bit of rest, added support and a nutritious diet.
- **Post-natal depression**: See below (up to 6 months after delivery).
- **Puerperal psychosis**: This is the most severe form, involving hallucinations and possible violence, usually dealt with as an inpatient in a specialist mother-and-baby psychiatric unit.

Post-natal depression may be brought on for several reasons:

- **Family history**: Sometimes there is a family history and the patient's mother suffered with a similar problem during the post-natal period.
- **Social**: It may be due to social circumstances, low finances, an unwanted child or lack of support from friends/family.
- **Hormonal**: There is no real theory to prove why, but some have proposed that it may be related to hormone levels, leaving some mothers particularly emotional during this period. So if it happens to a mother with her first baby she should be ready to expect something similar with subsequent births.

Key points

Counselling guidelines

As with all counselling stations, it is important to gain the patient's trust. Introduce yourself, be gentle, polite, smile if appropriate, make eye contact – all to show that you are trying to empathise with your patient.

Place importance on the mother initially and not just the baby

Ask:

- How she is feeling in herself?
- Is she eating and drinking well?
- When did she last go out with friends/shopping?

Find out about the circumstances surrounding the pregnancy

- Was the pregnancy planned?
- Are the family/partner supportive?
- How has it changed her life/job?
- Does she have any friends who have also become mothers recently, or does she feel isolated?

Find out how she is interacting with her new baby

- Were there any complications in the immediate post-natal period? Was she separated from the baby at any point? For how long?
- Is she breast-feeding the baby or bottle-feeding?
- Is she or her partner/friend changing the nappies?

Rule out any ideas of self-harm/harm to the baby:

- This is a difficult area to broach, but an important idea to rule out. You could subtly mention something like, 'Many mothers find it incredibly difficult during this period after delivery and want to give everything up, or sometimes want to give up the baby, have you ever felt this way?'
- Once you are happy the patient is not displaying ideas of self-harm or harm to her baby you can go on to advise her.

Management

First-line treatment for mild depression includes eating well, ensuring periods of rest for herself, regular contact with a health visitor and attendance at mother-and-baby groups where the patient can meet other women in similar circumstances.

If you feel the depression is a little more severe you can arrange for a regular community psychiatric nurse or social worker to visit her. This would allow someone to regularly assess her condition and make sure she is not deteriorating.

The last line of treatment would be to refer the patient to a psychiatrist for antidepressant treatment. Breast-feeding is fine with some of the newer tablets, but she should allow 4 weeks for the effects to be noticed. An outpatient follow-up appointment should be made after this time.

12

Assessing depression and suicide risk

Imagine you are the SHO covering for your consultant rheumatologist (who is currently water-skiing in the Bahamas!). A male patient with severe chronic gout has come in for a routine assessment. You have not met him before. You notice he looks a bit down and unkempt. Please take a history from this patient.

Answer follows . . .

Assessing depression and suicide risk

Answer

Most people will experience feelings of low mood and sadness at some point in their lives; however, at any one time 5% of the population will be clinically depressed. That is, they will have anhedonia, accompanied by symptoms such as impaired appetite, early morning wakening and diurnal mood variation, loss of concentration, loss of libido and slowness of cognitive functioning. There can also be ideas of guilt, worthlessness and hopelessness. Severe depression can lead to ideas of suicide and psychotic depression in which there are delusions and hallucinations. This section looks at how to take a competent history from a depressed patient.

Doctor–patient scenario

Dr T.: Hello Mr Low, I'm sitting in for Dr Tophi. How have you been since the last time we saw you?

MR L.: The pain's really been getting to me over these last few months.

DR T.: I'm sorry to hear that. Can you tell me a bit more about what's been happening?

MR L.: The pain's unbearable during the flare-ups, and even when it's down I find it hard to get myself up again.

DR T.: What do you mean by that?

MR L.: I just can't seem to get interested in anything anymore. All I can think about is the pain.

DR T.: What sorts of things have you lost interest in?

MR L.: I used to enjoy meeting the others at the pub for a few drinks every now and then, but I don't like leaving the house anymore. I find it hard to do anything nowadays – I can't seem to get motivated for anything. (*This is a fairly big clue to anhedonia, so you decide to look for other signs of depression.*)

DR T.: How's your appetite been recently?

MR L.: I used to enjoy my food, but since my wife died a couple of years ago I haven't been able to cook as much.

DR T.: Have you noticed any change in your weight?

MR L.: I reckon I may have lost a few pounds recently – my clothes seem to be a little looser.

DR T.: How have you been sleeping?

MR L.: Not so good – the pain keeps me up some nights, and other nights I wake up too early while it's still dark, and then I can't go back to sleep.

DR T.: OK. How do you feel once you're awake?

MR L.: I'm always tired, and I find it hard to get out of bed.

DR T.: Why is that?

MR L.: I ask myself, 'What's the point?' I don't have anything to do when I'm up. I do get out of bed later and I sometimes feel a bit better as the day goes on, but I feel a bit alone in the house so it's worse again by teatime. Each day is the same as the last – I have trouble remembering what day it is sometimes.

DR T.: Have you had any other problems with your memory?

MR L.: Like what?

DR T.: Like your concentration?

MR L.: I'm not sure.

DR T.: Do you find you can follow TV programmes?

MR L.: I lose interest quickly.

DR T.: OK. How long have you been feeling as low as you are now?

MR L.: It's been weeks now. I can't remember exactly.

(*The patient has many of the risk factors for being depressed – he is single, with poor social support, is getting older and suffers from a chronic debilitating condition. He shows the biological symptoms of depression. (Clinically, for him to be depressed, his symptoms must persist for over 2 weeks). You now ask questions to determine how severe his depression is.*)

Dr T.: Do you ever feel there's no point going on with life?

MR L.: I do sometimes wonder why I don't just finish it all. It's my fault I feel this way – there's no one else to blame.

DR T.: Have you ever tried ending your life?

MR L.: I did once – just after my wife died.

DR T.: It's sounds like her death affected you badly. How did you try to kill yourself?

MR L.: I took 48 paracetamol tablets and 48 'flu-tablets that I had at home.

DR T.: Do you remember the name of those tablets?

MR L.: No.

DR T.: OK, what happened after you took the pills?

MR L.: I woke up the next day feeling really rough, but it obviously hadn't worked so I called an ambulance.

DR T.: Did you actually want to die at that time?

MR L.: Yes, I was convinced it would work.

DR T.: Why did you choose tablets?

MR L.: They were in the house at the time.

DR T.: Did you need to stock up on them beforehand?

MR L.: No, they were all in the bottles.

DR T.: Right, did you write a suicide note?

MR L.: No.

DR T.: How did you feel afterwards?

MR L.: I felt stupid when I was in hospital.

DR T.: Why?

MR L.: I don't think it was the right thing to do. It's not right to kill yourself.

DR T.: Was that the first time you tried to harm yourself?

MR L.: Yes.

DR T.: Do you think you would ever consider it again?

MR L.: I don't think so.

Discussion

At this point you have enough information to make a risk assessment of future suicide intent. In this case the risk is low, as he seems to have no intention of trying again. Bear in mind that any new history of DSH (deliberate self-harm) should be referred for psychiatric assessment because up to 20% of people who attempt suicide will try again within 1 year; 1–2% of attempts will result in suicide.

Remember with any history of depression to rule out possible medical causes such as hypothyroidism, Cushing's disease, dementia, Parkinson's disease and so on.

13

Obtaining consent for autopsy

Mrs Carbona, a 64-year-old woman, suffered from endometrial carcinoma. A total abdominal hysterectomy and bilateral salpingo-oophorectomy was performed 7 days ago and she was recovering well after the operation. Yesterday, she died suddenly from a suspected pulmonary embolism. You were one of the doctors present at the resuscitation attempt. Take a consent to continue with autopsy from her next of kin, her son, Mr Carbona.

Answer follows . . .

Obtaining consent for autopsy

Answer

See also 'Breaking bad news' page 347. This is a very challenging station. It would be a difficult situation to approach at the best of times – the atmosphere needs to be quiet and private, and you need to spend a reasonable amount of time with the next of kin to be able to broach the subject in the appropriate manner, you yourself need to remain calm and controlled. The PLAB exam setting allows none of that!

The important thing to remember is that the person sitting in front of you in the exam will be an actor, and so it is your job to act along too.

- Always introduce yourself at the start of the session.
- Be empathetic, use understanding as a tool as opposed to sympathy.
- All people react to grief differently, be aware that you may face hostility.
- As with any other counselling station, explain the underlying principles of the situation in layman's terms, i.e. what a pulmonary embolism is, why an autopsy is done, etc.
- Get to the point sooner, rather than building up unnecessary anxiety.
- Remember to show respect and maintain eye contact; your body language should reflect a supportive attitude.
- At the end, ask if there are any questions and listen attentively.
- Thank the next of kin at the end of the session.

Doctor–patient scenario

Dr M.: Hello Mr Carbona, I'm pleased to meet you, my name is Dr M., I'm one of the doctors who was looking after your mother. We are all very sorry for your loss.

(*Offer to shake hands, but don't be put off if the actor declines a handshake at this stage.*)

DR M.: This is a dreadful time for everybody involved. How are you coping in yourself?

(*Actor may look away, remain stoical, laugh or cry.*)

DR M.: I realise this is a difficult time Mr Carbona, but I'd like to discuss an important and somewhat urgent matter with you today. However before I begin, do you have any questions for me, about anything at all?

MR C.: Why did she die?

DR M.: Mr Carbona, we think your mother suffered from a massive clot on her lung that compromised her lung function. This is a rare but serious complication of any pelvic surgery, and we had discussed this with her before her operation. Your mother underwent extensive surgery to remove the cancer and was in the operating theatre for a prolonged duration.

MR C.: So you killed her then. You are telling me this is a complication from your operation, something you knew would happen and you killed her!

DR M.: Not exactly. There is always a risk with any procedure. As we explained to your mother before her surgery, clots are associated with any long operation, particularly of the pelvic organs. It is very unfortunate that this happened, but it was not and could not be predicted or prevented. We tried our best to resuscitate your mother but unfortunately we were unsuccessful.

MR C.: What happened?

DR M.: Well, without further investigations we can only speculate on what happened to your mother over the past couple of days. Most probably it was a clot on her lung; however, we cannot be sure at this stage.

MR C.: How much longer will you take to be sure? She's

already dead for goodness sake.

DR M.: This is what I need to talk to you about Mr Carbona. When these situations arise it is very difficult for all involved, we feel that limitations in our knowledge have let us down. In situations where someone has died and we have questions about the cause of death, we recommend an autopsy to answer these questions. The only way to help rectify this for the future is to learn from such events.

(*No response from Mr Carbona.*)

DR M.: Just as you are suffering now, people have suffered before you, and until we as a medical profession know how to overcome this situation, others will continue to suffer after you. I understand that none of this will bring your mother back, although the information may be helpful to your family in the future.

MR C.: What are you saying doctor?

DR M.: I'm asking your permission, as next of kin, to forward your mother's body for autopsy. This is where a specially trained doctor will be able to further investigate what happened and confirm our suspected diagnosis, the clot on the lung. Sometimes the diagnosis is something different altogether, and the family is much relieved just knowing what really happened rather than living with an indefinite answer. Also, as I explained earlier, you don't feel it now, but you could be helping other people in the future.

MR C.: What does this autopsy mean? How will you investigate? Will you just do some blood tests?

DR M.: There will be tests involved. The body may be opened up briefly and investigated inside. Any scars will be on the trunk of the body, and they will be closed up for the funeral so that nothing will show.

(*No response from Mr Carbona. Maintain silence, allow him to have some thinking time.*)

MR C.: I don't think it's simply my decision doctor, all my

family is involved here. Can't you ask one of the others?

DR M.: You could discuss this with your family members, but you are legally the next of kin, and you have accepted this responsibility for your mother. The sooner we complete the investigation the sooner you will know, and may proceed towards the funeral. I appreciate that you would want to discuss this with your family. However, from a legal point of view, final consent is ultimately given by you.

MR C.: You are sure it won't delay the funeral?

DR M.: The sooner we begin, the sooner the investigation will be complete and you will know.

(*Silence from Mr Carbona, before continuing.*)

MR C.: I think it is important to know, I would like to know what happened to my mother. I think it's important to really know.

DR M.: It is a very difficult situation Mr Carbona, and it is your decision. Let me show you the consent form, so you may read what you would sign. Have you understood everything? Is there anything you want to ask me?'

(*If Mr Carbona should decide to give permission for the autopsy to go ahead, he must sign the form at the bottom. There is usually a space for the date, the name of the procedure to be conducted and your signature.*)

DR M.: Thank you, Mr Carbona, for your time and patience. (*Re-offer to shake his hand.*)

Note

Of course, when there is significant doubt as to the cause of death, when the death was not thought to be imminent, when the deceased had not been seen by a doctor within 14 days of their death, or when there is suspicion that death was the result of an accident, violence or neglect, the coroner will request an autopsy. In such cases, a family does not have to give consent, although they will always be informed.

9

Telephone conversations

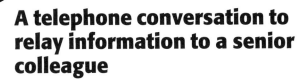

1

A telephone conversation to relay information to a senior colleague

Mrs Keeley had a right hemicolectomy and came back to the ward 6 hours ago. You are the surgical SHO on the ward when she suddenly collapses. The nurse brings Mrs Keeley's observation chart to you. Call your registrar and explain the situation over the telephone.

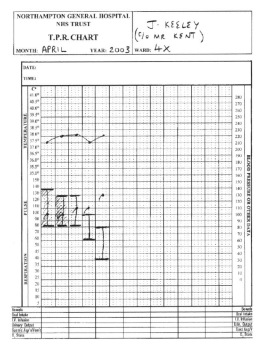

Figure 9.1 Observation chart showing a BP of 80/40 mmHg, pulse 130 beats/min, apyrexia, SpO$_2$ 100% on 10 L/min oxygen.

Answer follows . . .

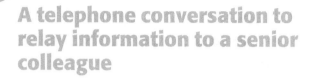

1

A telephone conversation to relay information to a senior colleague

Answer

Telephone conversations in the PLAB stations actually do take place over a telephone. You will be presented with a chart, and possibly other test results, and it is up to you to communicate them over the phone.

Whatever the situation, assess the basics – 'How is the patient's airway?' 'How is their breathing?' 'How is their circulation?' – and then apply your knowledge to the situation in hand.

SHO–registrar scenario

Hi Mr Kendrew, it's Dr H., the SHO on Ward 4X. I'd like to talk to you about one of Mr Kent's post-op. patients here.

The patient's name is Mrs Keeley, a 47-year-old woman, who underwent a right hemicolectomy 6 hours ago.

The case note written by Mr Kent suggests the hemicolectomy was performed for carcinoma of the caecum, with no metastases found in the liver/lymph nodes and no ascites.

She was in recovery for about 45 minutes and then brought to 4X where she was initially stable, until about an hour ago when her BP started dropping from 120/80 to 80/40. Her pulse rate has been gradually creeping up and she's tachycardic at 130/min right now.

On examination, her abdomen is distended and quite tense and tender. There's no evidence of any bleeding PR. Her chest is clear.

Her GCS has dropped from 15 to 11.

I'm treating her as an intra-abdominal bleed or anastomotic leak.

She has already been cross-matched from her previous Group and Save for a further four units of blood; I've put up a litre of Gelofusine (*Haemaccel or Hartmann's solution can also be used*).

She's already had a prophylactic dose of Clexane (*i.e. low molecular-weight heparin for the prophylaxis of DVT and PE*). Her calves seem soft on examination and her oxygen saturations were actually maintaining well on air. She's on high-flow oxygen at the moment. (*The airway is fine, you've ruled out a PE and DVT.*)

She received metronidazole and cefuroxime cover and is apyrexial (*rule out sepsis*).

Her repeat ECG shows no acute changes from previous tracings (*look for ischaemic changes such as a post-operative MI*).

Her gases (*arterial blood gases*) show a metabolic acidosis, pH 7.3, but her $p(O_2)$ and $p(CO_2)$ are within normal limits, her bicarbonate is 19 mmol/litre.

I've warned theatres there may be a patient for the emergency list, but I'd appreciate it if you would review her before going I go any further. Is there anything else you want me to do before you get here?

2

Meningitis

You are an SHO working in A&E. A mother has taken her child to the GP, who has diagnosed the child with an URTI. Mum is not satisfied, she is worried her child may have meningitis and has phoned A&E. Please take a history and reassure her.

Answer follows . . .

2

Meningitis

Answer

A telephone conversation is a difficult station to approach unless it has been clearly thought about beforehand. You should:

- Confirm the patient's ID over the phone.
- Remember to use the child's name to make the conversation more personal.
- Establish if other people are involved, e.g. other siblings, this is important.
- Give clear and comprehensive advice.

Doctor–parent scenario

DR M.: Hello, A&E department, this is Dr M. speaking, how can I help you?

MRS B.: Hello Dr M., my name is Cheryl Barter, I think my son has meningitis, I've been to see the GP who seems to think it's just a viral infection, I'm very worried.

DR M.: Alright Mrs Barter, don't panic, we'll talk through this together. To begin with could I check that I've got your name right and take your address and telephone number in case we need to contact you again?

(*Mrs B. confirms her name and gives you her address and telephone number.*)

DR M.: Thank you. And your son's name?

MRS B.: Tommy.

DR M.: Good, how old is Tommy?

MRS B.: He's three, doctor.

DR M.: Okay, tell me how this all started please.

MRS B.: Tommy went to nursery yesterday and he seemed quite tired when he came home. He didn't want his breakfast this morning. He seemed a bit lethargic so I didn't send him to nursery today, later on in the day his nose started running, he was sneezing and he was irritable.

DR M.: I see, well it certainly seems Tommy isn't 100% in himself. An important question Mrs Barter, have you noticed any rash on Tommy's body? Please go and check now.

MRS B.: No, there is no rash.

DR M.: Good, are you aware of the 'glass test' (*see 'Discussion', below*) Mrs Barter?

MRS B.: Yes, the GP explained it to me this morning. I understand about the glass test.

DR M.: Alright, how is Tommy at the moment, what is he doing?

MRS B.: He's playing with some toys; he isn't too irritable at the moment.

DR M.: Please observe him playing, is he enthusiastic or drowsy? Is he using all his arms and legs, moving his head and neck as usual?

MRS B.: Well, I suppose he's quite enthusiastic at the moment! He seems to be playing like he normally does.

DR M.: Okay, that's good. Have you taken his temperature, does Tommy feel as though he has a fever, is he complaining of feeling cold?

MRS B.: No there is no temperature, doctor.

DR M.: Have you given Tommy any Calpol or Junifen already?

MRS B.: No I haven't yet, I wanted to speak to you first.

DR M.: Sure. Is Tommy sitting by the window or is the light on. Have you noticed if Tommy is aggravated by bright light in any way?

MRS B.: Well, the room is adequately lit, as normal really.

He seems okay with it.

DR M.: Good. I know Tommy is very young, but has he complained of a headache?

MRS B.: He was irritable previously, but he hasn't mentioned anything since then.

DR M.: Has Tommy been sick at all?

MRS B.: No, but he didn't eat any breakfast this morning.

DR M.: Do you have any other children Mrs Barter? How are they?

MRS B.: I have a daughter, aged 7. She's been fine, she's at school at present.

DR M.: Good, Mrs Barter, I also do not think Tommy has meningitis for the following reasons. Tommy does not have a rash on his body, he does not have a temperature, he is playing normally at present displaying no neck stiffness which is often a key sign in meningitis. He isn't having any difficulty with light, another sign, and you feel he is back to much his normal self. I think this may well be a viral infection and I would go ahead and give him some Calpol. However, I can appreciate your concern, so please continue to keep an eye on him, look out for the signs we talked about, and also keep an eye out for any skin rash. Remember to try the glass test. Watch for any vomiting or if Tommy becomes very drowsy or very irritable.

MRS B.: Yes, thank you doctor, I will.

DR M.: You can always go back to your GP, or contact us again if necessary. Of course, you can always bring Tommy to the hospital for a check if you're still worried.

MRS B.: That's great, thanks again.

DR M.: You're welcome, goodbye Mrs Barter.

Discussion

In reality, the conversation might not go quite as smoothly! The child might have a rash somewhere that the mother is unsure about; or, more than likely, the child would be pyrexial and bit off colour. If in doubt, you would always ask to see the child for yourself.

Never just give advice over the telephone if you are not sure.

Why did you ask about other siblings?
It is important to ask about siblings/other family members to establish any mode of contact.

If you decided this could be meningitis, what further action would you take?
I would establish if Mrs Barter had transport to bring Tommy to the hospital, immediately. If not, an ambulance/alternative transport would be arranged so that Tommy could be brought to A&E for assessment.

If confirmed as meningitis, I would notify my senior doctor and probably the paediatric on-call doctor for a fast-track admission.

If a fast-track admission was not possible, I would attempt iv access and give an immediate dose of a cephalosporin antibiotic at the correct dose for the child. Along with iv fluids, I would make regular observations/neuro-observations and take blood samples.

What is the 'glass test'?
This is a simple test that helps to educate the public with regards to a purpuric rash. Pressure is applied to the rash by rolling a clear glass over it. If the rash disappears (blanches), it is non-purpuric. If the rash remains and can still be seen through the glass (non-blanching), it is likely to be a purpuric rash, which may be a case of meningitis and needs to be further assessed by a professional.

Informing a patient of a missed diagnosis

You are the SHO in A&E, you have just received a phone call from the reporting radiologist that a patient you sent home yesterday, complaining of pain in her left hip, actually has a fracture of the neck of her femur. These things happen, but the most important next step is to call the patient back to hospital for admission, informing her of the missed fracture.

Answer follows . . .

Informing a patient of a missed diagnosis

Answer

Doctor–patient scenario

DR S.: Hello there, I'd like to speak with Ms Hobbis please.

MS H.: Yes, speaking.

DR S.: Oh, hello there Ms Hobbis, I'm sorry to bother you, this is Dr S., calling from St Elsewhere hospital, we met in A&E yesterday.

MS H.: Oh, what a surprise! Well I'm glad you called, I still have an atrocious pain in my hip and the pain killers really aren't helping a jot!

DR S.: Well that's why I'm phoning today Ms Hobbis, a little bit of bad news I'm afraid. The X-ray I took of your hip yesterday, which I'd initially thought was clear, was re-reviewed today, and it appears that there may actually be a fracture . . . a break in the bone there.

MS H.: Oh! Well, that's a shock!

DR S.: Yes, I'm very sorry I didn't see it yesterday. But it certainly seems there may be a break there, and I think we need to get you seen by the specialist bone doctors as soon as possible. Would you be able to come back to us straight away?

MS H.: Do I really need to come all that way again? Can't my GP take things from here now you know what's the matter?

DR S.: I'm afraid it isn't as simple as that, you may need to be admitted onto a ward. Again I apologise for the inconvenience Ms Hobbis, but if you have somebody to drive you here I think it might be wise to get you seen as soon as possible.

MS H.: I see. Well, my husband can bring me. Should I bring my night-clothes?

DR S.: I think that would be a good idea. You're taking things very well, I'm most grateful, and again I apologise I didn't see the fracture yesterday.

MS H.: Well, you've been very good to me so far, and I know you were trying your best. Anyway, I'm glad you've found something wrong to put right, because this pain is just unbearable!

DR S.: I imagine you must be in terrible pain. As soon as you get here, we'll give you some stronger pain relief and get you seen. Thank you for your co-operation Ms Hobbis, I'll come and see you myself as soon as you get here.

MS H.: Okay then. I'll ask my husband to pack a case. Goodbye.

DR S.: Goodbye, see you soon.

Discussion

These things happen! And they will continue to happen.

In the above conversation, being courteous, explaining the situation to the patient and admitting that a mistake has been made seemed to have kept the patient in an agreeable mood.

These are tricky situations and the patient has every right to be angry, but the most important thing is to rectify the situation calmly and efficiently.

4

Relaying information to a relative

Mrs Callaghan is an inpatient in the elderly care unit; she has been admitted this morning acutely confused ?cause following admission to the Medical Admissions Unit. You have only just reviewed her on the ward round and are about to request a number of investigations.

Miss Callaghan, daughter and the next of kin of Mrs Callaghan, is on the phone asking how her mother is doing and what the next step of treatment is likely to be. Please talk to her.

Answer follows . . .

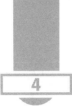

4

Relaying information to a relative

Answer

Doctor–relative scenario

DR M.: Hello, my name is Dr M., I'm the doctor on the elderly care ward. May I confirm who I'm speaking to please?

MS C.: Oh, hello doctor. I'm Miss Callaghan. I believe you're looking after my mother, she was admitted last night, could you please tell me what's wrong with her?

DR M.: For purposes of confidentiality Ms C., as I'm sure you'll appreciate, I'd like to take your telephone number and check against our records that it is correct. I can then phone you back. Is that alright?

MS C.: Oh, well I suppose so.

DR M.: I'd also like to check with Mrs Callaghan that she is happy for me to talk with you. Please don't take this personally Ms C, it is routine practise and for the benefit of the patient.

MS C.: No, not at all.

DR M.: OK, could give me your number?

(Ms C. gives her telephone number.)

DR M.: Right, we'll get back to you as soon as we can. In the meantime, do you have any other questions?

MS C.: Will, I have to wait long?

DR M.: No, I understand you must be concerned for your mother. It won't be long.

MS C.: OK, thank you doctor.

DR M.: Goodbye

DR M.: Hello there Ms C., thank you for waiting for me to return the call. I have just spoken with your mother. What can I help you with?

MS C.: What is the matter with my mother?

DR M.: When she came to us yesterday, she was quite dehydrated and a little confused. She has lost a considerable amount of weight recently and so it's important for us to rule out any sinister causes for her presentation. We have put her onto a drip, which has certainly helped her to pick up. However, her blood tests revealed her calcium level was high, which may have caused both the dehydration and confusion, and this is a matter we need to address with some urgency.

MS C.: I see. Why should my mother suddenly get this? Is it something that was always there and wasn't picked up by her own doctor?

DR M.: Not necessarily. There could be a number of causes for the calcium level to be raised, we need to investigate the various possibilities.

MS C.: Like what?

DR M.: I wouldn't want to speculate; but with the history of weight loss, we do need to rule out any sinister underlying problems.

MS C.: Like cancer?

DR M.: A malignancy is just one of the many things that could present this way. We're waiting for the results of the investigations and hopefully these will help us understand exactly what has happened to your mother, and how best to treat her.

MS C.: Doctor, may I ask something?

DR M.: Of course.

MS C.: A lot of my aunties and uncles have had cancer of the bowel. I think it must run in the family. They all lost weight too. If it is cancer, please don't tell my mum just yet, I don't think she'll be able to handle it. It's probably best if you tell me or my brother. We could break the news to her.

DR M.: I know you're very concerned for your mother, but I'm afraid I can't promise anything. Your mother has a right to know, and if she asks me, I will tell her as much as she would like to know. But if she says she doesn't want to know, we won't tell her. It's important to us that she has that choice though. Again, once we make a diagnosis, whatever it may be, it is only with your mother's permission that I can relay this information to yourself or any other family member.

MS C.: She'll break down if you tell her something like that. I know my mother.

DR M.: I appreciate what you are trying to tell me, and I am grateful for the warning. If the diagnosis is cancer, we do have special nurses, Macmillan nurses, who will be able to talk to and counsel your mother very delicately and with great dignity. If your mother should ask, I do not feel I can withhold information from her.

MS C.: But doctor, look perhaps I'm not making myself clear. Would you speak to my brother he's just here, he can explain things better than me.

DR M.: I understand, but I don't really feel it's appropriate to conduct such a conversation over the telephone. If you are willing, I'd be happy to speak to both of you on the ward in person.

MS C.: Okay. I'll be coming during visiting hours today. Could I speak to you then?

DR M.: I should be on the ward and I'll be happy to speak with you. Thank you for understanding; I look forward to meeting you. Goodbye.

MS C.: Thank you, doctor. Goodbye.

Discussion

Talking over the phone to relatives is something that is

done on a daily basis. As a healthcare professional you can be put on the spot. It is important to remember the following key points:

- Always establish and attempt to confirm who you are speaking to.
- You may only give information to a relative if you have obtained the patient's permission.
- In complicated scenarios, it is probably more confidential and will cause less confusion if you call the relative onto the ward for a discussion.
- Always be polite and adopt a professional attitude.
- Telephone conversations, particularly with relatives who are pressurising you, can be difficult, but it is important to maintain patient confidentiality and respect at all times.
- If you are asked questions you are unable to answer adequately, stop, explain you are not entirely informed at present. Ask for senior help if necessary.

Appendix 1

Question bank

The PLAB, Part 2 OSCE examination consists of actual OSCE stations, one rest station and one 'pilot' station. A total of 12 stations are included in each examination; each station will last for 5 minutes and a bell should ring at 4 minutes 30 seconds, giving the candidate time to 'close up'.

This appendix contains two mock OSCE examinations, compiled from remembered past questions set by the GMC.

Mock OSCE examination – 1

1. Ms Walkden is a 30-year-old woman complaining of pain in the right upper quadrant. Please take a history from her, perform an abdominal (not GIT) examination and arrive at a possible diagnosis.

2. Mrs Boulton has come to the gynae outpatient clinic for a routine cervical smear (*anatomical model would be used*). Please proceed to take a cervical smear, fix and label it.

3. You are the senior house officer on night duty working on the Graham Steelle ward, no other staff are presently available. You suddenly hear a loud noise from an adjacent cubicle, upon entering the cubicle you find one of your male patients lying on the floor. What would you like to do in this scenario?

4. Mrs Stephenson, a 50-year-old woman, has been complaining of a severe headache for the past few days. Please take a relevant history and explain the nature of her underlying illness to her.

5. Mr Jennings is a 73-year-old man with known metastatic carcinoma of the colon. He is suffering from abdominal pain despite taking regular paracetamol and co-proxamol. He has been admitted to the oncology ward for pain relief. How would you tackle this problem and further advise this patient (mention what analgesic you might use and any side-effects you would like to notify the patient about)?

6. Mrs Patel is 48-year-old woman who has recently been started on diuretic treatment. She is presenting to you

complaining of dizziness. Please measure her blood pressure.

7. A 20-year-old woman, Miss Bonita, has come to you very tearful and feeling depressed; she gave birth 4 weeks ago and is finding it difficult to cope with her new baby. Please talk to this new mother and discuss your plan of action for her.

8. Mr Peterson has brought his 5-year-old son, Christopher, to your clinic. Christopher has recently been diagnosed with asthma, please teach him how to use his inhalers (salbutamol and Flixotide).

9. You are the SHO in A&E, Mrs Brown has phoned you for advice, her 3-year-old daughter, Kelly, woke up unwell this morning, and has not been feeling well since. Mrs Brown is worried this may be meningitis. Please take a history from her and advise her accordingly.

10. Please obtain an informed consent from a patient advised to have a herniorraphy for a left-sided inguinal hernia.

11. Mr Gitelman, a 35-year-old businessman, has recently returned from the Far East. He has been suffering with diarrhoea for the past 4 days, and is feeling unwell. Please take a history from him and arrive at a list of possible diagnoses.

12. Mr Liddle is a 60-year-old man who was thrombolysed for an anterior MI. His recovery was uneventful and he is now ready for discharge. You are the SHO working on CCU, please advise him on what lifestyle changes he needs to make post-MI.

Mock OSCE examination – 2

1. Mr Pallman presents to you with a history of fresh PR bleeding. Please take a relevant history and confirm a diagnosis.

2. Mrs Petrie has come to you for advice regarding HRT, please counsel her.

3. You are the SHO in A&E, a man (builder, identity not confirmed) has fallen from a rooftop. Please assess his Glasgow Coma Scale. (GCS chart provided.)

4. Mrs Saha is a 26-year-old lady (manikin available) who is due to go theatre as an emergency for an ectopic pregnancy. Please ascertain iv access and take blood samples for relevant pre-operative investigations/requirements.

5. Mr Reynolds is a 46-year-old man who is on a skiing holiday in the Alps; he is complaining of severe knee pain. You are the local doctor, please perform a knee joint examination. (Actor present.)

6. Mrs Barter has brought her 16-year-old daughter to you, Trisha, who has been losing a lot of weight recently. Mrs Barter is concerned, please take a history from Trisha and establish a list of differential diagnoses.

7. Miss Angelman is an 18-year-old college student who has recently been diagnosed with epilepsy, please counsel her about lifestyle changes appropriate to her condition.

8. Mr Jeffrey is a known IDDM, he presents to you in clinic for an annual check-up. Please talk about what you would like to do.

9. Mr Birey is 59 years of age, and has presenting to you with a history of recurrent chest infections and shortness of breath (COPD). Please conduct a respiratory examination and show him how to use a peak flow meter.

10. This is an ECG of a 58-year-old man presenting with chest pain, in resuscitation – A&E. Interpret the ECG (anterolateral MI), and discuss your immediate management.

11. A 35-year-old woman with three children has come to the outpatients gynaecology clinic with her husband, requesting tubal sterilisation. Counsel and advise her regarding this request.

12. You are shown an abdominal X-ray, which shows dilated large bowel loops. The nurse tells you this patient has been constipated over the past 5 days and is complaining of abdominal pain and vomiting. What further questions would you like to ask the nurse. What are the possible causes for this type of abdominal film?

Appendix 2

Colloquialisms/ euphemisms

Dictionaries of slang are available for most regions/counties of the UK.

3 sheets to the wind	drunk
40 winks	short nap/sleep
6 feet under	dead/feel very unwell
acid	lysergic diethylamide (LSD)
aggro	aggressive trouble/troublemaking (abbrev. of aggravation)
alcohol	booze, grog (specifically rum), gut-rot, hard-stuff, jar, moonshine
all the rage	fashionable
ants in pants	restless/fidgety
argy-bargy	dispute/wrangle, especially a loud quarrel
arse	buttocks
arse-hole/ass	anus/term of contempt for a person
away with the fairies	senile
B.O.	body odour
back passage	anus
back-door	underhand/clandestine/anus
bairn	small child (generally in NE England and Scotland)
balls	testicles
banged up	imprisoned/sexual intercourse

bark up the wrong tree	wrong assumption
bathroom	can just mean a toilet
bawling	loudly crying child
beak	nose/law judge
beer-gut/-belly	protruding belly attributed to excessive beer drinking
belch	loudly emit wind from the stomach through the mouth
belly	abdomen
belt up	admonition to stop talking
big C	cancer
bird	woman
black out (verb; blackout, noun)	to lose consciousness (e.g. to faint or fit), vision, memory
bloomers	women's underpants
blow his/her top	'explode' in rage
blub	cry
blues, the	depressive episodes, usually post-partum
bog	toilet
bonce	head
boobs/boobies	breasts
booze	alcoholic drink
bosoms	breasts
bread	food/money
brood over	worry about
bubbly	champagne/sparkling personality
bum	buttocks/derogatory term for a person/beggar
bum-steer	false information
bunged up	blocked
burp	see 'belch'/to make a baby belch by, e.g., rubbing its back
bust	breasts/broken
butt	buttocks
C	illicit cocaine
cat's whiskers	an excellent person/thing
cat on hot bricks/ tin roof	in a state of agitation
catnap	short sleep

catty	sly/spiteful person
charlie	illicit cocaine
cheers	now used as a general term for 'thank you'
chip off the old block	child resembling a parent, esp. in character
choke	impede breathing/disappointed/upset
chops	the jaw/cheeks (facial)
chow	food/type of dog
churn up	state of agitation
clammy	unpleasantly moist/damp/sticky feeling/humid atmosphere
clap	gonorrhoea
clobber	clothes/criticism/to hit a person
clock	face
cock	penis/term of endearment/friendship
codger	person, usually an old person
coke	cola drink/ illicit cocaine
collywobble/s	strong feeling of apprehension/rumbling or pain in the stomach
conk	nose
conk out	to break down/become exhausted/die
consumption	tuberculosis
crabby	perverse/bad-tempered
crabs	pubic lice
crack	illicit free-based cocaine
crack up	mental breakdown
crackpot	eccentric person
crap	faeces/nonsense/rubbish
creeps	nervous feeling
crick	sudden onset of stiffness in the neck or back
crinkle	wrinkle ('a crinkly', an old person)
croak	deep, hoarse voice/die
cropper, to come a	fall heavily/fail badly
crotchety	peevish/bad-tempered
dick	penis
dilly-dally	dawdle/vacillate
dinner	main meal of the day, either around mid-day or in the evening
dither	indecision/tremble
dizzy	vertiginous/silly person

doddery	tremble/totter/unsteady due to old age
dog	canine/unattractive woman
dog's breakfast/dinner	messy
dog's life	a life of misery
dog-tired	exhausted
dope	illicit drug/information
dose	venereal disease
dotty	eccentric person
double-Dutch	incomprehensible talk
down below	external genitalia/buttocks area
drop off	fall asleep
dump	defecate
E	the drug Ecstasy
eye-opener	revelationary experience/an alcoholic drink to start the day
fag	homosexual person/cigarette
fanny	female genitalia
fart	emit wind from the anus
fed up	depressed
fiddlesticks	nonsense
finicky	over-particular/fussy
firing blanks	absence of sperm
fits and starts	spasmodically
fits, in	laughing uncontrollably
flabbergasted	greatly astonished
flap, in a	in a state of agitation
flummoxed	bewildered/confused
fly off the handle	sudden and unexpected loss of temper
frog in the throat	hoarseness
front botty	external genitalia
funk/blue funk	fear/panic/coward
funny bone	elbow
gaffer	a boss/old person
gag	retch
gaga	senile
gammy	lame/injured
ganja	cannabis
get it up	penile erection

giddy	vertiginous feeling/excitable or frivolous person
gift of the gab	extremely voluble
gip/gippy tummy	diarrhoea/upset stomach
glasses	spectacles
gnashers	teeth
gob	mouth
gone/going to the dogs	deteriorate
grass	cannabis
green around the gills	feeling of nausea
green	cannabis
gripe	complain/gastric or intestinal pain
grog	alcoholic drink (originally rum)
groggy	unsteady/shaky, not necessarily caused by alcohol
gross	large amount/horrible
grub	food
gut-rot	alcohol
guts	intestines/a brave person
gutted	devastated
guy	man
guzzle	consume greedily
H	illicit heroin
hacking cough	short, dry frequent cough
hair of the dog	another alcoholic drink to cure the effects of drink
half cock	unready ('go off at half cock', strongly react before all information has been given)
hammered	drunk
hanker	want
hard on	penile erection
hard stuff	alcoholic drink
hash	cannabis
have a fit	greatly surprised or outraged
haywire	erratic/out of control
head	toilet
heartburn	indigestion
henpeck	harass/pester
herb	cannabis

higgledy-piggedly	disorganised/disorderly/muddled
hitched	married
Hobson's choice	no choice
hooch	alcohol
horse	illicit heroin
hotchpotch	jumbled mixture
huff/huffy (in a huff)	annoyed/take offence
hum	noise made with the mouth closed/bad smell
icky	sweet/sticky/sickly smell/taste/feeling
iffy	uncertain/doubtful
innards	intestines
insides	stomach and bowels
itch	sexual desire
ivories	teeth
jabber	chatter volubly (sometimes means to talk incoherently)
jar	alcoholic drink
jaw	chatter volubly
jellies	illicit vallium
john	toilet
john thomas	penis
joint	cannabis cigarette
jump on	attack or criticise a person
keel over	fall over
kibosh	nonsense ('to put the kibosh on', to stop something happening)
kick in the teeth	a humiliation
kick the bucket	die
kid	child
kip	sleep
kisser	mouth
knackered	exhausted
knocked up	sexual intercourse
knockers	breasts
lass/lassie	young girl
lather, in a	in a state of agitation
lav/lavatory	toilet
lead in my/his pencil	penile erection
legless	drunk, especially too drunk to stand upright

let the cat out of the bag	divulge a confidence
line, a	illicit cocaine
loaf	to laze around
long in the tooth	old
loo	toilet
lose his/her marbles	show symptoms of senility
lose his/her rag	lose his/her temper
losing it/lost it	show symptoms of senility
lost the plot	show symptoms of senility
lughole	ear orifice
magic mushroom	mushroom producing psilocin, a hallucinogen
manky	dirty/inferior
mitts	hands
Montezuma's revenge	diarrhoea
mop	hair/implement for cleaning floors
mug	face
muppet/mup	silly person
mush	mouth/face/soft pulp
mushies	magic mushrooms
namby-pamby	weak/insipid person
nan/nana	grandmother
nancy	homosexual man
nap	short sleep
natter	chatter volubly
needle	annoy
nerves	stress/anxious ('got a nerve', impudence)
nipper	small child
nippy	quick/nimble/cold/chilly
nit	silly person
nit-picking	petty fault-finding
nits	head lice
no sweat	no trouble/bother to do something
nobody home	alone in the house/senile person/derogatory term
nod off	go to sleep
noodle	head
noggin	head/small measure of drink
nooky	sexual intercourse

nosh	food
not all there	a person who is senile or who has learning difficulties/also used in the derogatory sense
nowt	nothing
number 1	urine
number 2	faeces
nut	head/testicles/to hit someone with your head
off his/her trolley	demented
on the ball	alert
out of sorts	slightly unwell
pain in the arse/backside/neck	troublesome person/thing
palaver	fuss and bother
pang	sharp pain/qualm/an emotion
pansy	homosexual man
pass out	faint/lose consciousness
pate	head
pecker	mouth
pee	urine
peepers	eyes
peg	leg
peg out	die
percy	penis ('point percy at the tiles', urinate)
period	menses
perished	died/worn out/feeling of intense cold
pernickety	over-precise or fastidious person
physog	face
pickled	drunk
piddle	urinate ('piddling', small, meaningless thing)
pie-eyed	drunk
piffling	small, meaningless thing
pig-out	over-eat
pill	contraceptive pill/the drug ecstasy
pins	legs
pins and needles	tingling sensation
pins, on	state of anxiety/trepidation
piss	urine ('take the piss', to mock)

pissed	drunk
plates (of meat)	feet
pong	bad smell
poo	faeces
poof	homosexual man
pooped	stool/tired
pop his/her clogs	die
porkie	a lie/untruth
posterior	buttocks
pot	cannabis
pox	venereal disease
prick	penis
private parts	genitalia
privy	toilet
puke	vomit
puss/y	female genitalia/a cat
put the boot in	commit an adverse physical or mental act upon another person
quack	doctor
queen	homosexual man
queer	homosexual man
reefer	cannabis cigarette
rest room	toilet
rocker, off one's	demented/also used in the derogatory sense
roly-poly	plump
rule out	exclude
rum	odd event/thing/person
runs	diarrhoea
schnozzle	nose
screw	sexual intercourse
seedy	unwell
shag	sexual intercourse/tobacco
shattered	exhausted
shilly-shally	indecision
shit	exclamation of disgust/defecate/ urinate/worthless person
short fuse	quick temper
short, taken	incontinent
shut your face	admonition to stop talking

skag	illicit heroin
skunk	a variety of cannabis
slap and tickle	light-hearted amorous event
slap on the back	congratulations
slap on the wrist/in the face	mild reprimand
slapdash	careless and hasty
slash	urinate
slipshod	careless/slovenly
slithery	slippy
slobber	saliva running from the mouth/show excessive sentiment
sloshed	drunk
smack	illicit heroin
smalls	underclothes
smart	stinging pain
smoke	tobacco or cannabis
sniffy	disdainful
snog	kiss
snooze	short sleep
snow	illicit cocaine
sopping (wet)	drenched
sorted	okay/resolved
sozzled	drunk
special K	trade name of a breakfast cereal/illicit ketamine
specs	spectacles
speed	amphetamine used as illicit drug
speedball	illicit cocaine and heroin mixture for injection
spend a penny	go to the toilet
spew	vomit
spittle	saliva
spliff	cannabis cigarette
spout, up the	ruined/hopeless/pregnant
sprog	child or baby
squidgy	squashy/soggy
squiffy	slightly drunk

squit	small or insignificant person/nonsense/diarrhoea
starchy	over-precise/prim person
starving	state of hunger/feeling of cold
stew, in a	anxious state
stewed	drunk
stitch in the side	acute pain in the side of the abdomen
stitched up	betray
stomach it	tolerate
stomach-ache	pain in the abdomen (not necessarily confined to the stomach)
stoned	under the influence of alcohol/drugs
streetwalker	prostitute
stuffed	satiated/blocked
supper	light meal before bedtime
sweat about, in a	in an anxious state
tab/s	tablet, generally LSD
taken from me	died
tanked up	drunk
tea	meal around 5–6 pm
tenterhooks, on	anxious state
thatch	hair
the curse	menses
thick	person with learning difficulties/derogatory term
thick-skinned	insensitive person
thingumajig/thingummy	used when a person has forgotten (or doesn't wish to use) the correct word
throw up	vomit
time of the month	menses
tipple	alcoholic drink
tits	breasts
tizz/y	in a state of agitation
toad	repulsive person
tomboy	a young girl who behaves like a boy
topsy-turvy	muddled/disorganised/disorderly
toss/tosser	male masturbation/derogatory term for a person
tot	small child/measure of alcohol

trap	mouth
trip	drug-induced hallucinatory state/journey/stumble
trots	diarrhoea
trotters	feet
tuck/er	food
tummy	stomach/abdomen in general
turd	faeces/derogatory term for a person
twaddle	nonsense
twist my/his/her arm	apply coercion, especially mental pressure
vegetarian	some 'vegetarians' eat fish, some also eat white meat
wank/er	masturbate/derogatory term for a person
water	urine
waterworks	urinary system
wc	abbrev. for water closet, i.e. toilet
wee/wee-wee	urine
weed	cannabis
well-oiled	under the influence of alcohol
whiffy	smelly
whinge	whine/grumble
willy	penis
wimp	person who is ineffectual or weak/also used as a derogatory term
windbag	person who talks a lot, generally about nothing
wishy-washy	insipid thing or person
with-it	fashionable
wolf down	eat greedily
women's problems	gynaecological problems
woozy	dizzy/unsteady/slightly drunk
worry-guts	a person who habitually worries unnecessarily
wrecked	exhausted/drunk
X	illicit drug ecstasy
yack	chatter volubly
yucky	disgusting/nauseous
zit	pimple

Index

Further reading

Collier, J.A.B. et al, 1995. *Oxford Handbook of Clinical Specialities*, 4th edition, Oxford University Press.

Dornan, T. & O'Neill, P., 2000. *Clinical Skills for OSCEs in Medicine*, 1st edition, Churchill Livingstone.

Feather, A. et al, 1999. *OSCES for Medical Undergraduates*, Vols 1 & 2. 1st edition, PasTest Ltd.

Impey, L., 1999. *Obstetrics and Gynaecology*, 1st edition, Blackwell Science.

Lissauer, T. & Clayden, G., 1996. *Illustrated Textbook of Paediatrics*, 1st edition, Mosby.

Molloy, D.W. et al, 1991. *American Journal of Psychiatry*. Volume 140.

Wasan, R. et al, 2000. *Radiology Casebook for Medical Students*, 1st edition, PasTest Ltd.

Useful websites

www.bbc.co.uk/health

www.bhsoc.org (British Hypertension Society Guidelines)